# ATTAINMENT'S

# Memory TIPS

## FOR MAKING LIFE EASIER

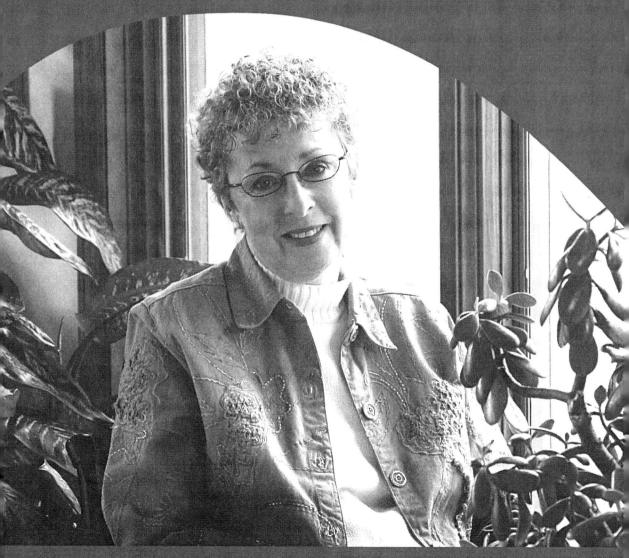

## Shelley Peterman Schwarz

**Memory Tips for Making Life Easier**

By Shelley Peterman Schwarz

Edited by Tom Kinney and Elizabeth Ragsdale

Graphic design and illustration by Elizabeth Ragsdale

Photography by Beverly Potts

ISBN: 1-57861-572-0
An Attainment Publication
©2006 Attainment Company, Inc. All Rights Reserved.
Printed in the United States of America.

**Attainment Company, Inc.**
P.O. Box 930160
Verona, Wisconsin 53593-0160
1-800-327-4269
www.AttainmentCompany.com

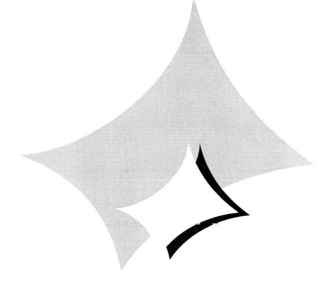

# contents

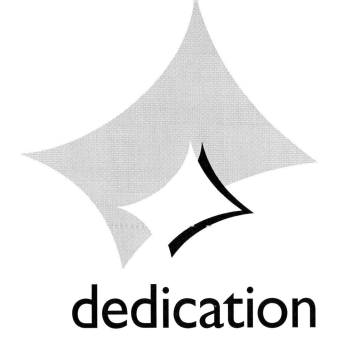

# dedication

To Judy Ross, my mentor, cheerleader and dear friend:
Thank you for believing in me!

To Ina Sharkansky, my quiet, unwavering supporter:
Thank you for your kindness and friendship.

To Deborah Proctor, my right arm and able assistant:
Thank you for all your hard work!

To my husband, David: There are no words to
adequately thank you for giving me the freedom to
live my life to the fullest. YOU are a remarkable man!

To all my wonderful friends and neighbors:
Please know that I couldn't do what I do without
you, and you have my deepest, heartfelt thanks.

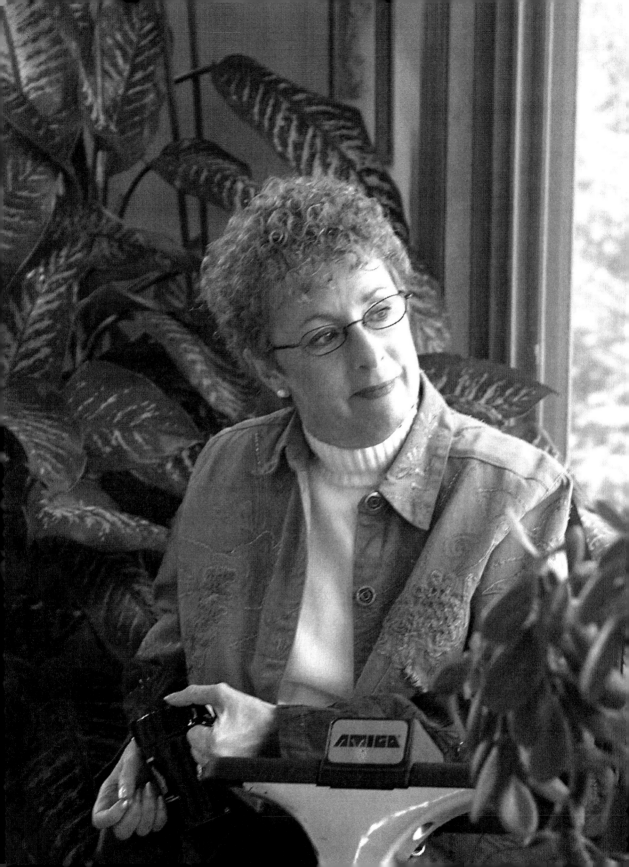

# introduction

**Dear Readers,**

I don't know if it's my age or if my life is busier than it used to be, but I'm forgetting things—like why I went into the freezer, what I was going to tell my best friend, where the car was parked at the shopping center or how to retrieve voice mail on my cell phone. It's not the big stuff of life but often the little things that makes one question, "Is my memory going?" It certainly helps when colleagues, coworkers, friends and family members empathize and say the same things happen to them.

While this book is intended for those wanting to improve their memories, people who have significant memory loss are unlikely to read this book. But family members and caregivers can pass these tips along to the end user.

If you are a healthcare professional, a family caregiver, a person feeling the effects of aging or just someone overwhelmed with all the things that must be remembered, this book is written for you. It will give you ideas you can use today to exercise your brain, remember more and feel confident that you haven't forgotten something.

The information in this book was gathered from three sources: (1) interviews and observations of people like you who are juggling lots of tasks, (2) my personal experience living with multiple sclerosis (MS)—an illness that often causes cognitive problems, and (3) my involvement as a long distance caregiver to aging in-laws.

**Memory Tips for Making Life Easier** features:

- Hundreds of tips and techniques
- Ideas for lists and charts you can create
- Unique products, services and resources and how to locate them

If you are a caregiver, what is the best way to administrate all these ideas? First, keep yourself healthy, exercise your brain and practice a few general memory techniques (see Chapter 1—Basic Concepts).

At the beginning of each chapter, you'll find insights and observations I've made in the process of writing this book.

Following this introduction is a section for assessing needs. Assessments allow the reader, whether end user or helper, to take a quick inventory of needs. Note that the assessment pages precede the actual tips, so you may want to scan the tips for further information. However, the assessment lists are self-evident and you should be able to fill out most of them without reading the tips first. Don't hesitate to scan the tips first, though, if you find it helpful.

It's my hope that the concepts, suggestions, strategies and ideas in each chapter will help you remember more; feel more comfortable dealing with people who have a memory loss; and find services, resources and products to assist you.

To help you get the most from this book, I've used Helping Hands and Advanced Memory Loss symbols to designate tips especially for caregivers:

**Helping Hands:** Tips for caregivers who assist people with mild cognitive problems.

**Advanced Memory Loss:** Tips for caregivers who assist people whose judgment, communication and daily living skills have been seriously affected.

If, after reading this book, you would like to share your own Making Life Easier tips, I can be reached at http://www.MakingLifeEasier.com and help@MakingLifeEasier.com.

**All the best,**

*Shelley*

**Shelley Peterman Schwarz**

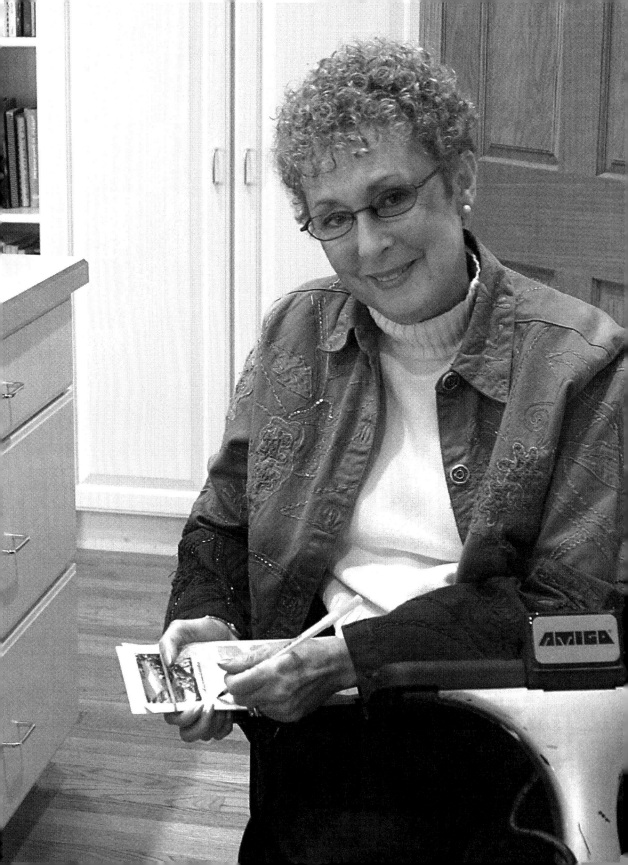

# basic concepts

The older I get, the more I realize that life will always be busy. No matter how old I am, I will always need to keep track of, remember and recognize people, places and things. My memory will always be taxed to keep dates straight, appointments scheduled, deadlines met and more.

As the years go by, it's likely that I will also have to help others remember the details of their lives. It helps me to rely on a few basic concepts. I'm sure some of these observations will be familiar to you. Others might be timely reminders. After you read through the basics, you'll be better able to integrate the information in the following chapters to improve your memory.

# ASSESSING YOUR NEEDS

**To create a healthier lifestyle, it would be helpful to:**

- ○ Cultivate a positive attitude
- ○ Eat and drink a healthy diet
- ○ Breathe deeply
- ○ Slow down and concentrate
- ○ Relax
- ○ Get enough sleep
- ○ Keep things in perspective
- ○ Set limits and boundaries
- ○ Ask for help
- ○ Be evaluated for depression

**To keep my brain active, it would be helpful to:**

- ○ Exercise my body regularly
- ○ Exercise my brain with creative activities
- ○ Do things differently
- ○ Stay actively involved in social activities
- ○ Learn new things
- ○ Understand my learning style
- ○ Pay attention
- ○ Be an active listener
- ○ Use all my senses

**To remember better, it would be helpful to:**

- ○ Do it now
- ○ Write it down
- ○ Visualize
- ○ Create rhymes and tunes
- ○ Make up stories
- ○ Develop acronyms
- ○ Make associations
- ○ Group like items together
- ○ Divide information into manageable pieces
- ○ Walk backward in my mind

**To provide support, it would be helpful to:**

- ○ Guide choices
- ○ Provide a relaxed and stable environment
- ○ Make the home environment safe
- ○ Establish rituals and routines
- ○ Use memory aids
- ○ Experiment with new approaches

# A healthy lifestyle

**Cultivate a positive attitude.** Attitude is everything. Having a positive attitude makes you more alert and receptive to receiving and remembering information. Believe you have a good memory and you will be more likely to relax and recall information.

• • • • • • • • • • • • • • • • • • • • • • • • • • •

**Tell yourself you will remember.** Your mind does not differentiate between positive or negative thoughts. It only knows what you tell it. Prepare for success and tell your mind what to do.

• • • • • • • • • • • • • • • • • • • • • • • • • • •

**Eat, drink and remember.** Protect and nourish your brain cells by eating a diet rich in fruits and vegetables. And—you've heard it before—drink water. A lack of water leads to dehydration, which can leave you feeling tired and unable to concentrate. To make sure you get enough water, fill four 16-ounce bottles in the morning and sip on them throughout the day. Keep a bottle in strategic places—on your desk, by the bed or where you watch TV—and carry one with you.

• • • • • • • • • • • • • • • • • • • • • • • • • • •

**Breathe deeply.** Several times a day, practice deep breathing exercises. Here's how: Relax and exhale completely through your mouth. Then, through your nose, draw in a deep breath—you should feel yourself sitting or standing taller. Hold this breath for a few seconds to allow your body to absorb all the oxygen and then exhale through your mouth again, making an audible sound. Repeat this pattern three more times. As your brain receives more oxygen, you will likely find that you think better and remember more. As an added bonus you may even find yourself sitting and standing taller.

• • • • • • • • • • • • • • • • • • • • • • • • • • • •

**Slow down and pay full attention.** Normal aging changes the brain and may make your mind slightly less efficient. Though you may lose some capacity for new memory as you age, experience compensates for this loss. Forgetfulness may indicate nothing more than having too much on your mind. Slow down and pay attention to the task at hand.

• • • • • • • • • • • • • • • • • • • • • • • • • • • •

**Relax.** Stress and anxiety can interfere with concentration, so it's important to take time to relax. Practice deep breathing, contract and relax each muscle in your body one at a time or take a virtual escape by closing your eyes and imagining yourself on a beach or other relaxing place. Just 10 minutes a day can make a positive difference in your abilities.

• • • • • • • • • • • • • • • • • • • • • • • • • • • •

**Encourage sleep.** A good night's sleep is an important key to a good memory. Try to establish going-to-bed rituals that are calming—away from the noise of television, meal cleanup and active family members. Exercise, limit caffeine during the day and discourage daytime napping to help prevent nighttime restlessness.

• • • • • • • • • • • • • • • • • • • • • • • • • •

**Keep your perspective.** You're not the only one who's placed a coffee cup on the roof of your car and driven away or dialed a telephone number only to forget whom you're calling. It happens. Take note of it, but unless you feel it's unusually frequent, don't be concerned. Everyone has difficulty remembering things at times. Try to focus on how much you do remember rather than what you don't.

• • • • • • • • • • • • • • • • • • • • • • • • • •

**Know your limits.** Overextending yourself, whether at work or play, can have detrimental effects on your body. Increased stress from too much to do and aches and pains from overdoing make it harder to concentrate and remember. If you find yourself forgetting things, take a look at your lifestyle. Can you simplify it by eliminating nonessential activities?

• • • • • • • • • • • • • • • • • • • • • • • • • •

**Tell your family and friends** how they can help instead of fretting about forgetting things. Tell them to watch you write down a scheduled event. If you haven't written it down, they should assume you have forgotten it and call to remind you well in advance. They might also be enlisted to help you remember to take your medicine, keep track of appointments, get chores done or get dressed. We can all make life easier if we ask for the help we need and allow ourselves to accept help from those who love us.

. . . . . . . . . . . . . . . . . . . . . . . . . . .

**Deal with depression.** If you feel sad, sleep poorly, don't enjoy eating, lack energy or have lost your sense of humor, you may be depressed. See your doctor to find out whether you have clinical depression. When treated, you will feel much better and will engage, interact and remember better.

# Exercising your brain

**Exercise your mind** by exercising your body. People who exercise briefly each day will be more alert and quicker mentally. Exercise results in improved strength, flexibility, endurance and cardiovascular health. It can also improve energy, circulation and mood. For people with memory difficulties, exercise can impart a sense of meaning or purpose and create a calming effect. Chances are, if you're exercising regularly, you'll sleep better too— another key to keeping your mental powers in shape.

. . . . . . . . . . . . . . . . . . . . . . . . . . .

**Choose a leisure activity** that exercises your right (creative) brain. Leave the logic and planning behind and act on instinct. Doodle, view or create art, listen to or make music. Even pinball, juggling or Nintendo are good right brain activities because they force you to act instinctively.

• • • • • • • • • • • • • • • • • • • • • • • • •

**Do things differently.** Anything out of the ordinary will give your mind a welcome workout. Try reciting tongue twisters, memorizing short poems or wise sayings, and reading aloud or upside down.

• • • • • • • • • • • • • • • • • • • • • • • • •

**Keep your brain active.** Read, write letters, keep a journal or diary, sing, dance, whistle, paint or draw and stay involved in social activities.

• • • • • • • • • • • • • • • • • • • • • • • • •

**Learn new things.** Challenge yourself with word games and puzzles, stay informed about the world around you and try new things. Go online or enroll in an interesting class; learn a new language, hobby or musical instrument; make a new friend; become a volunteer. Learning new things will add new brain cells and strengthen memory connections.

• • • • • • • • • • • • • • • • • • • • • • • • •

**Know your learning style.** Matching your memory strategies to your learning style will help you remember better. Do you learn better by seeing or hearing? If you don't know, try this little test. Have someone watch your eyes as they ask you familiar questions: "How much is 2 plus 2? Where do you live? What is your pet's (spouse's, child's) name?" Then have them ask you a question that requires some thinking: "Where did you go on your last vacation?" If you looked at the ceiling before you answered, you are a visual learner. If you looked to the side (toward your ears), you are an auditory learner. Using several senses at once, of course, will increase your ability to remember.

● ● ● ● ● ● ● ● ● ● ● ● ● ● ● ● ● ● ● ● ● ● ● ● ● ● ● ●

**Pay attention.** Many times we forget things like names, dates and times because we're not paying full attention when the information is shared. Make a conscious decision to "listen up."

● ● ● ● ● ● ● ● ● ● ● ● ● ● ● ● ● ● ● ● ● ● ● ● ● ● ● ●

**Be an active and engaged listener.** When you take an interest in the subject, you're more likely to remember details, facts, sequences and events.

● ● ● ● ● ● ● ● ● ● ● ● ● ● ● ● ● ● ● ● ● ● ● ● ● ● ● ●

**Use all your senses** to keep your memory sharp. Multiple cues such as silky bathrobe (touch), calming aromatic herbs (smell), soothing music (hearing) and a sign on the door or the light from an open doorway (sight) could all be cues for getting ready for bed. Be careful, however, not to overdo the stimulation and cause added confusion.

## General memory techniques

**Do it now.** This is probably the most important memory enhancement technique. If you act immediately, you have no need to remember.

• • • • • • • • • • • • • • • • • • • • • • • • • • •

**Write it down.** Write notes, make lists, create "cheat sheets" and construct timelines.

• • • • • • • • • • • • • • • • • • • • • • • • • • •

**Visualize.** Form a picture in your mind. Use your imagination to add humor, action or exaggeration.

• • • • • • • • • • • • • • • • • • • • • • • • • • •

**Create rhymes and tunes.** Use rhyming words or create new words for familiar tunes to help you remember tasks, sequences, dates and facts.

• • • • • • • • • • • • • • • • • • • • • • • • • • •

**Make up stories.** Link items together in your mind by putting them in story form. (Remember how story problems helped you learn math?)

. . . . . . . . . . . . . . . . . . . . . . . . . . . . .

**Develop acronyms.** Using the first letter of each item you want to remember, create an acronym or funny phrase such as KISS (Keep It Simple Stupid).

. . . . . . . . . . . . . . . . . . . . . . . . . . . . .

**Make associations.** Relate new information to something you already know.

. . . . . . . . . . . . . . . . . . . . . . . . . . . . .

**Group like items together.** Organize your mind like a grocery or department store, with similar items or categories all in the same aisle.

. . . . . . . . . . . . . . . . . . . . . . . . . . . . .

**Divide and conquer.** When learning something new, break up the subject into manageable sections and concentrate on one section at a time.

. . . . . . . . . . . . . . . . . . . . . . . . . . . . .

**Retrace your steps mentally** to retrieve a thought, remember where you left your coffee cup, remind yourself what you were looking for or recall what you wanted to do next.

. . . . . . . . . . . . . . . . . . . . . . . . . . . . .

**Encourage correct choices.** If a loved one has difficulty knowing where things are or where to go, look for ways to use simple modifications and visual cues to help guide decisions. Add a nightlight in the bathroom to make it easier to find; paint or decorate the door to the bedroom so it's distinctive from other doors; put pictures of eating utensils, dishes, towels and food items on the outside of cabinets and drawers. Little things can go a long way in helping a loved one with memory loss be more independent.

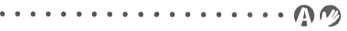

**Provide structure for stability in the home.** Anxiety can result from new situations, noise, large groups of people, being pressed to remember or being asked to do a task that's too difficult. As anxiety rises, the ability to think clearly declines.

**Make the home familiar and safe.** When memory is an issue, keeping everything in the same place is an important strategy. To help prevent accidents around the home, install locks on cabinets containing medicines, toxic substances and dangerous utensils or tools; remove electrical appliances from your bathroom; set the water heater no higher than 120° F; and install grab rails.

**Avoid the urge to change** the way things are done. Establish rituals for everything from getting dressed to going to bed at night.

• • • • • • • • • • • • • • • • • • • • • • 🅐🖐️

**Use memory aids** to help a friend or family member remain independent. Write out a list of the day's activities, telephone numbers to call for help and instructions on how to do simple tasks such as make a cup of tea or use the telephone.

• • • • • • • • • • • • • • • • • • • • • • 🅐🖐️

**Try a new approach.** If a technique you've used before stops working, be flexible, patient and understanding as you try to find a solution.

• • • • • • • • • • • • • • • • • • • • • • 🖐️

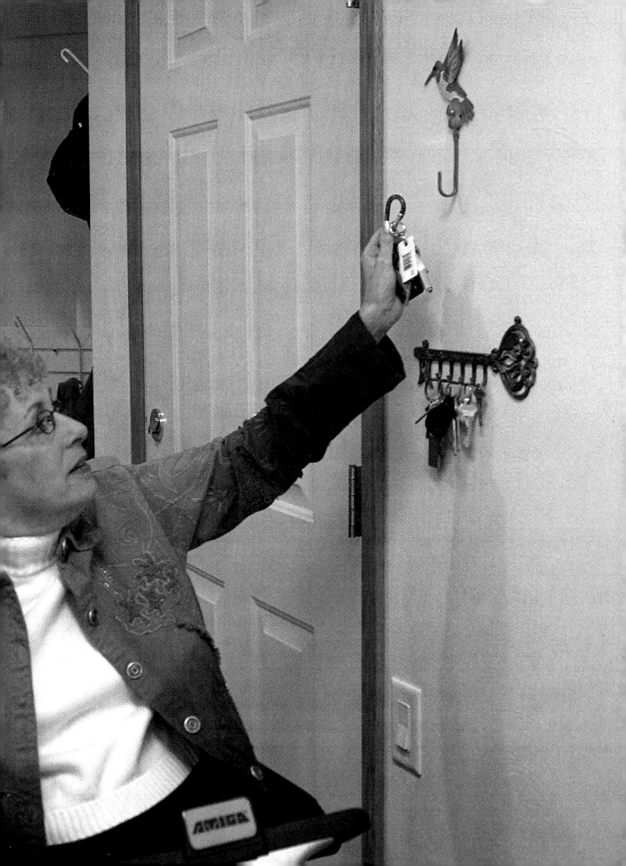

# 2

# strategies
# for living

Where did I leave my keys? What did I do with the
directions for retrieving voice mail? How can I possibly
remember all the rules to the game of bridge?
Whenever we find a strategy that helps us tackle one
of life's challenges, our memory improves and we feel
empowered to handle more. This chapter offers ideas
for taking charge of your life. I hope they help you.

# ASSESSING YOUR NEEDS

**To get organized, it would be helpful to:**

○ Have a specific place for everything
○ Have duplicate items for different rooms
○ Gather things together in containers
○ Store tools on a pegboard
○ Create a photo mobile
○ Use color-coded holders

**To organize papers, it would be helpful to:**

○ Use a Homeowner's Record Keeper
○ File appliance manuals and warranties
○ Use three-ring binders with pockets
○ Keep important documents in containers
○ Use color-coded clipboards and step files
○ Use a card file box for addresses
○ File or store by category
○ Store tips and articles in folders
○ Store magazines in plastic bins
○ Attach reminder notes with binder clips

**To establish a routine, it would be helpful to:**

○ Complete tasks in the same order
○ Make a to-do list before going to bed
○ Plan daily activities at the beginning of the week
○ Organize my week using daily to-do baskets
○ Use a monthly organizing system

**To develop good habits, it would be helpful to:**

○ Keep a diary
○ Log telephone calls
○ Use appointment books, planners and calendars
○ Write tasks on 3" x 5" cards
○ Make notes In book margins or on business cards
○ Make duplicate notes with carbonless paper

**To use lists to remember, it would be helpful to:**

○ Write realistic to-do lists
○ Organize myself for the next day
○ Keep a checklist in every bag

**To help remember what I'm doing, it would be helpful to:**

○ Practice repetition
○ Tell myself what I'm doing as I'm doing it
○ Set up object cues
○ Put greeting cards next to unpaid bills
○ Count the number of items I'm taking with me
○ Make a note indicating where I stopped
○ Group monthly chores together

# ASSESSING YOUR NEEDS

**To simplify things, it would be helpful to:**

- ○ Simplify tasks by breaking them down
- ○ Remember steps to the whole
- ○ Use color coding
- ○ Hide things where I'll remember them
- ○ Arrange for monthly bill paying assistance
- ○ Sort mail to direct attention to the most important things

# Get organized

**Always return items to specific places.** Hang keys on a hook by the door. Clip your cell phone to your belt or put it in a specific pocket in your purse. Place eyeglasses in a case on your nightstand. Tuck sunglasses in your car visor. Put credit cards in the same slot in your wallet.

• • • • • • • • • • • • • • • • • • • • • • • • •

**Purchase duplicate items** and keep them where they're used. Buy a pair of scissors for every room (kitchen, bathroom, office, kids' rooms, den). Have extra soap and toilet paper in every bathroom and a full set of cleaning supplies on every floor. Keep an extra pair of reading glasses where you most often use them. Nannini Flat Specs Readers, available in a wide array of colors and five magnifying strengths, fold flat and come with their own tiny case. About $18. Per Annum Inc., 48 W 25 St., 10th Floor, New York, NY 10010; 800-548-1108; www.flatspecs.com.

• • • • • • • • • • • • • • • • • • • • • • • • •

**Gather things together.** Put a basket, box or plastic bin near the door you use most often when you leave your house. Use the container to hold items you need to remember to take with you the next time you go out. When you're ready to go, everything, including purse and car keys, is waiting at the door. If the load is awkward to carry, you can use the container to transport the items to the car.

• • • • • • • • • • • • • • • • • • • • • • • •

**Store tools on a pegboard.** Use a marking pen to outline the space for each tool. It will help everyone remember where the tool goes and indicate at a glance if a tool is missing.

• • • • • • • • • • • • • • • • • • • • • • • •

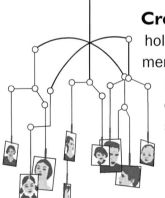

**Create a mobile** out of favorite photographs, holiday cards or children's artwork. Keep memories in sight and in mind with the Kikkerland Photo Mobile. Clips at the end of each stainless steel arm hold just about any size photo or card, attractively displaying your collection in very little space. About $14. Exit9, 64 Avenue A, New York, NY 10009; 212-228-0145; www.shopexit9.com.

• • • • • • • • • • • • • • • • • • • • • • • •

**Use color-coded holders** in your purse or briefcase. If you are always losing things in your purse, purchase different colored holders coded to the contents (e.g., credit card holder in chocolate brown, glasses case in green, makeup bag in maroon and change purse in cherry red).

• • • • • • • • • • • • • • • • • • • • • • • •

# Organize your papers

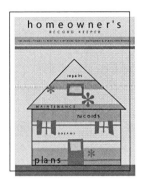

**Keep track of household repairs,** maintenance, projects, plans and dreams with a Homeowner's Record Keeper. This workbook provides a quick reference to key contacts, maintenance checklists, tip sheets for hiring professionals and room by room decorating logs, as well as space for swatches of material, paint or wallpaper. About $19 at Chronicle Books; www.chroniclebooks.com.

• • • • • • • • • • • • • • • • • • • • • • • •

**Keep household appliance manuals** and warranties in a special file. If you have misplaced a manual, go to www.appliance411.com for links to over 30 manufacturers and online versions of manuals. You will find information such as how microwave ovens work and how to avoid calling a repair person.

• • • • • • • • • • • • • • • • • • • • • • • •

**Use three-ring binders with pockets** to organize your household papers. Use separate binders for recipes, car maintenance records, home maintenance documents, warranties, health club schedules, classes and medical information.

• • • • • • • • • • • • • • • • • • • • • • • •

## Keep important documents in containers.

Store receipts, bills, warranties and so forth in clear or colorful plastic pouches, accordion files, folders or binders. Once a month go through your receipts and file large-purchase credit card receipts by company so you'll know where to find them if you need to return something. Toss unneeded cash receipts and shred ATM, deposit and credit receipts after checking them against your statements. If you keep your filing system up to date and labeled with the same categories used on income tax forms, doing your taxes will be easier.

● ● ● ● ● ● ● ● ● ● ● ● ● ● ● ● ● ● ● ● ● ● ● ● ● ● ● ●

## Use color-coded clipboards and step files.

Things out of view are often forgotten. One way to keep to-do lists and other important information orderly and in view is to store color-coded clipboards in a stepped file holder, which displays folders at different heights. Use a different color (pink = office, blue = business, green = household) for each category or family member. Step files store neatly on your desk or countertop and are easily seen and accessed. Viking and Reliable are two manufacturers of step files, which can be found at most office supply stores.

● ● ● ● ● ● ● ● ● ● ● ● ● ● ● ● ● ● ● ● ● ● ● ● ● ● ● ●

**Use a card file box for addresses.** Instead of the usual address book, purchase a 3" x 5" card file box, index cards and alphabetical index tabs. You'll have space to write all the things you want to remember in one place: Names, addresses and phone numbers, work numbers and addresses, anniversaries and birthdays. A Rolodex file, available from office supply stores, keeps telephone numbers handy. When people move, it's easy to replace their card.

• • • • • • • • • • • • • • • • • • • • • • • • • • •

**File or store by category.** If you have trouble remembering the specific names of businesses or agencies you need to contact on an occasional basis, record or file this information first by category and second by the letter of the alphabet. For example, file doctors by specialty or put all telephone information (equipment and service providers) in one general "telephone" category.

• • • • • • • • • • • • • • • • • • • • • • • • • • •

**Store tips and articles** in categorized folders. If you tend to keep magazines around for that special article, recipe, craft project or decorating idea, and then can't remember where to find what you're looking for, try cutting out the things you want to save and recycling the rest. Sort recipes by type, articles by topic and craft projects by kind, season or topic. Store in folders for each category so you'll be able to find what you're looking for quickly and easily.

• • • • • • • • • • • • • • • • • • • • • • • • • • •

**Store old magazines in clear plastic bins** so you can remember what's inside. If you store them by month rather than title, it'll be easier to find things like seasonal recipes or project ideas.

• • • • • • • • • • • • • • • • • • • • • • • •

**Attach reminder notes with binder clips.** Available at office supply stores, binder clips can be used on baskets, shelves, the visor of your car—anywhere you need to keep a note handy. You can even hang a clip from a hook or refrigerator magnet, allowing you to keep an assortment of notes together for easy access.

# Establish a routine

**Creating good habits** allows your memory to work on only the important things. You can develop a routine for almost everything, from getting ready in the morning to how you drive home. Then even on the most stressful days, your mind will walk you through your daily routine as if on autopilot.

• • • • • • • • • • • • • • • • • • • • • • • •

**Complete tasks in the same order** and store keys, glasses, purses or wallets in the same place so you know where to find them. If you tend to forget your bag when you're out, put it in front of you where you can easily see it and are less likely to leave it behind.

• • • • • • • • • • • • • • • • • • • • • • • •

**After dinner or before bed,** organize yourself for the next day by gathering up all the materials you'll need for your errands. Put everything by the door or in the car for the following morning.

**Structure the daily routine** to maintain a sense of familiarity. Not only will this help a person remember where to go or what to do next, it will help others locate the person if need be.

**Write down step-by-step instructions** for tasks performed infrequently. Use pictures to illustrate the tasks and post the steps near where the activity is performed so everyone can follow the instructions easily. This will provide continuity of care and reduce confusion for the person with memory problems.

**Establish a calming nighttime ritual** away from the noise and activity of other family members. During the day limit caffeine, promote exercise and discourage napping.

**To keep from being overwhelmed,** make a list at the beginning of each week of what you need to accomplish. Use a daily planner or wall calendar. Break the list down to no more than one difficult or time consuming task per day. If you think you might not get everything done, prioritize your list. If a task remains undone, add it to the next week's list.

• • • • • • • • • • • • • • • • • • • • • • • • • • • •

**Dedicate a basket or shelf** to each day of the week to help you remember what to take with you each morning. Place things on the shelf or in the basket for the appropriate day. When you leave that day, you'll have all the things together you need.

• • • • • • • • • • • • • • • • • • • • • • • • • • • •

**Monthly organizing system.** To help you remember what needs to be done tomorrow, next week or next month, try this: Take 11 manila folders with tabs across the top. Using a yellow highlighter, color 5 tabs and write one weekday on each tab, alternating the position of the tab. Use an orange highlighter on the next three folders and write "1 Week," "2 Weeks" and "3 Weeks" on them. Color the last three folders with a green highlighter and label them "1 Month," "2 Months" and "3 Months." Place paperwork in the appropriate folder. if something is not finished at the end of the day, transfer it to the next day's folder. At the end of the week, move all the remaining tasks to the appropriate folder for the following week.

• • • • • • • • • • • • • • • • • • • • • • • • • • • •

# Develop good habits

**Write it down.** If you start working on one task and something else pops into your head, write it down on a piece of paper, your personal data assistant (PDA) or calendar. Studies have shown that if you write things down, you're 100%–200% more likely to remember the item or complete the task.

• • • • • • • • • • • • • • • • • • • • • • • • •

**Keep a diary** so you can recall what you did, who you talked with and so forth.

• • • • • • • • • • • • • • • • • • • • • • • • •

**Log telephone calls,** recording the date and time of the call, the person you spoke with and what you discussed. Not only will this help imprint the information in your memory, but you'll have a permanent record of the conversation should you need to refer to it later. A telephone log can be extremely helpful when you communicate with technical support, billing departments, insurance companies and Social Security.

• • • • • • • • • • • • • • • • • • • • • • • • •

**Use appointment books,** planners and calendars to organize your schedule. (See Chapter 4: A Matter of Time.)

• • • • • • • • • • • • • • • • • • • • • • • • •

**Use a spiral or steno notebook** to keep all your notes and reminders in one place. Keep a small pen or pencil handy in the spiral binding.

• • • • • • • • • • • • • • • • • • • • • • • • •

**Write tasks on 3" x 5" cards.** Refer to the cards periodically during the day, while you're on the phone, waiting at a stoplight or even sitting at a meeting, to remind yourself of what you need to do. Reuse cards for frequent tasks.

• • • • • • • • • • • • • • • • • • • • • • • • •

**Jot notes in the margin.** When reading for business or pleasure, keep track of main points, characters, anything you might want to remember later by making notes in the margin. Notes are especially helpful for a novel with a complicated cast of characters or foreign names.

• • • • • • • • • • • • • • • • • • • • • • • • •

**On the back of a person's business card** write down where you met, something about the individual's appearance, what you talked about—anything that will jog your memory later.

• • • • • • • • • • • • • • • • • • • • • • • • •

**To remember what you said in a note,** use carbon paper between two sheets of notebook paper and keep the copy. You can also use carbonless paper available by the sheet or ream at office supply stores.

• • • • • • • • • • • • • • • • • • • • • • • • •

# Make lists

**Write realistic to-do lists.** Rather than making a long list you'll never be able to complete, include only two or three things if this is all you can handle or have time to do in a day. When you accomplish everything on your to-do list, you'll feel more in control of your life and less stressed.

• • • • • • • • • • • • • • • • • • • • • • • • • •

**Before you go to bed,** make a to-do list for the next day and put it in your purse so there's no chance that you'll leave home without your list.

• • • • • • • • • • • • • • • • • • • • • • • • • •

**Keep a checklist** in every purse, bag or backpack. Then it's easy to remember everything you need.

# Use repetition and cues

**Practice repetition.** To help remember a person's name, work it into conversation several times. Repeat a list of things to do several times or create a little rhyme or song to help you remember.

• • • • • • • • • • • • • • • • • • • • • • • • • •

**Tell yourself what you are doing** as you're doing it. For example, say out loud: "I'm locking the door." "I'm putting the dishes away." "I'm turning off the light." By increasing the number of senses involved in any activity, you increase your ability to remember.

• • • • • • • • • • • • • • • • • • • • • • • • • •

**Set up cues.** For example, put items you need to take with you by the door.

• • • • • • • • • • • • • • • • • • • • • • • • • •

**Use object cues.** This technique is similar to tying a string around your finger. For example, turn your ring or watch around, put a crumpled bill in with your change or tip a lampshade. Noticing something different will remind you that you're supposed to remember something. Review the association often so you don't forget what the changed object represents.

• • • • • • • • • • • • • • • • • • • • • • • • • •

**Put birthday and anniversary cards** next to your unpaid bills. When you pay the bills, you'll remember to mail the cards too.

• • • • • • • • • • • • • • • • • • • • • • • • • •

**Count the number of items** you're taking with you. When you leave the house or are traveling, count the number of items you're taking with you (e.g., umbrella, purse, raincoat and scarf = four items). When you move from place to place, count your items before you leave to make sure you remember everything you came with. Or count the parts of your body (hands, head, shoulders and toes) to remember your mittens, hat, coat and boots.

• • • • • • • • • • • • • • • • • • • • • • • •

**Write a note indicating where you stopped** work on a project, whether for a short interruption or a longer period. Use a sticky note and add comments that will help you get back on task quickly and easily.

• • • • • • • • • • • • • • • • • • • • • • • •

**Associate monthly chores** with other monthly activities. If you want to remember to do monthly chores like changing air conditioner filters or giving the dog his heartworm pills, associate them with other monthly rituals like paying the telephone bill.

• • • • • • • • • • • • • • • • • • • • • • • •

# Simplify things

**Simplify tasks** by breaking them down into easily identifiable, sequential steps.

• • • • • • • • • • • • • • • • • • • • • • • • •

**Remember steps to the whole.** If you have trouble remembering information, break it down into parts. Tell yourself what happened first, then next. Or try to remember just two things. Once you have the framework, your memory can build on what you know.

• • • • • • • • • • • • • • • • • • • • • • • • •

**Use color coding.** For example, purchase yellow twin sheets and white queen-size sheets or blue tablecloths for one table leaf and red cloths for two leaves. Assign a different colored basket to each family member or day of the week. Color-code your contact lenses by ordering one colored and one clear to help remember which lens goes in which eye.

• • • • • • • • • • • • • • • • • • • • • • • • •

**If you hide something for safekeeping,** don't be too creative. You may have difficulty remembering your hiding place. When you leave on a trip, for example, put your extra jewelry in the out-of-season winter boots you're leaving at home. If you do forget where you put the jewelry, come winter, you'll find it.

• • • • • • • • • • • • • • • • • • • • • • • • •

**Arrange for monthly bill paying assistance.**
If you have trouble remembering to pay your bills, ask your bank to send a clerk to your home once a month to help with bill paying or recordkeeping. Some banks offer this service at no charge.

• • • • • • • • • • • • • • • • • • • • • • • • •

**Sort mail into three categories:** Needs Action, Toss and Read Later. Then you can direct your attention to the most important things first.

• • • • • • • • • • • • • • • • • • • • • • • • •

**Create a reorder system for office supplies.**
When you purchase new cartridges, attach a sticky note to the last cartridge. The note should include reorder information such as type of machine (copier, fax, printer), location, reorder number, quantity usually ordered and any other pertinent information. This system can also be used for office and home supplies.

• • • • • • • • • • • • • • • • • • • • • • • • •

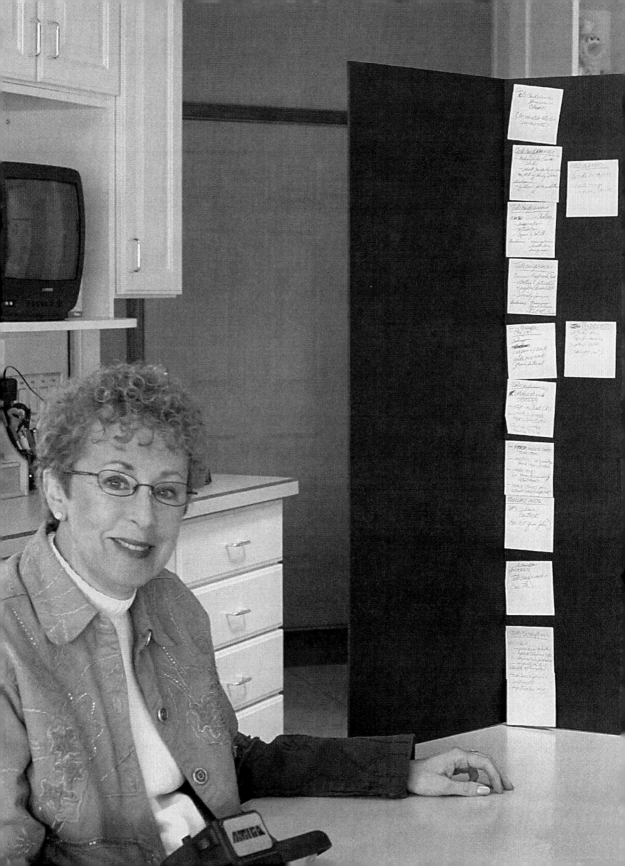

# 3

# the little
# details of life

It's easy for me to get upset and frustrated with myself when I forget someone's name, phone number or birthday. And yes, it's comforting when friends say, "That happens to me, too." However, I get tired of making excuses, getting embarrassed and feeling like "I'm losing it." To regain control over these minor lapses in memory, I've used the memory tips and aids in this chapter many times. I hope they'll also help you remember all the little details in your life.

# ASSESSING YOUR NEEDS

**To remember everyday details, it would be helpful to:**

- ○ Visualize
- ○ Create mental pictures
- ○ Make associations
- ○ Group like items
- ○ Use acronyms, funny phrases, rhymes and alphabet cues

**To remember names, it would be helpful to:**

- ○ Use repetition
- ○ Spell names in my head
- ○ Link names to place or occupation
- ○ Create a mental picture
- ○ Use association or word pictures
- ○ Rhyme names
- ○ Review names of attendees
- ○ Ask for help remembering names
- ○ Use a sense of humor

**To remember dates, it would be helpful to:**

- ○ Associate information with a date
- ○ Create a rhyme or song
- ○ Use prices or times for dates

**To remember numbers, it would be helpful to:**

○ Keep a list of frequently dialed telephone numbers
○ Say numbers out loud
○ Create words to remember phone numbers
○ Look at the pattern created when dialing the phone
○ Make up a song for a phone number
○ Enter phone numbers on a calculator
○ Use cell phone features

**To use the telephone more easily, it would be helpful to:**

○ Get free directory assistance
○ Take note of automatic phone menus
○ Use a cordless phone
○ Use an Amplified Photo Phone
○ Mark the "0" on the phone
○ Put an address and phone label on the phone for emergencies
○ Use a Telephone Hanger-Upper

**To find things more easily, it would be helpful to:**

○ Breathe deeply and count to 10 when something is lost
○ Walk backward in my mind
○ Put car keys with items I want to remember
○ Keep container of essentials in the glove compartment
○ Mark possessions I tend to lose

# ASSESSING YOUR NEEDS

**To use sticky notes to remember, it would be helpful to:**

○ Write sticky note reminders and post where needed

○ Use sticky notes to indicate action needed on each item of a project

○ Remember errands with sticky notes

○ Use eye-catching sticky notes

○ Keep a sticky note with my PDA

**To use lists to remember, it would be helpful to:**

○ Shop with a list

○ Keep a list of phone numbers by the phone

○ Keep a list of doctors and medications in my wallet

○ Make a list of questions for the doctor

○ Make lists that can be used over and over again

○ Create a permanent packing list

○ Make a list with sticky notes

**To use high tech and low tech aids to remember, it would be helpful to:**

○ Set an alarm as a reminder
○ Remind myself with a vibrating locket
○ Program a pager with reminders
○ Program numbers into the cell phone
○ Use a personal data assistant
○ Tape record reminders
○ Record step-by-step instructions
○ Leave a message on the answering machine
○ Take digital pictures
○ Use the NetPost CardStore to send greeting cards

**To use a computer to remember, it would be helpful to:**

○ Create a WHERE.IT.IS file
○ Set the computer alarm
○ Send myself email messages
○ Write down access codes
○ Keep passwords in a dummy folder
○ Use one access code for everything
○ Keep computer glasses at the computer
○ Use the AutoCorrect feature
○ Use the Bookmark feature
○ Search with Google

# Mental pictures and word games

**Visualize what you want to remember,** such as day of the week, where you will be, what you will be doing and who you will be with. Imagine yourself in that location, on that day, doing what you will be doing. When the time comes, you'll be more likely to remember. You can use this technique to remember appointments, names or when to take your medications.

• • • • • • • • • • • • • • • • • • • • • • • • • •

**Create a mental picture.** If you suffer from intermittent memory lapses, like forgetting a name or particular word, tell yourself not to fret about it. Relax and create a mental picture of what you want to remember. If you are going to the grocery store to pick up five items (e.g., chicken, milk, bread, bananas and laundry detergent), think of a chicken washing clothes while eating a banana sandwich with milk. The crazier the mental picture, the better.

• • • • • • • • • • • • • • • • • • • • • • • • • •

**Link things together.** Salt and pepper, cats and dogs, day and night—these are things always associated with each other. Make up your own associations to remember names or items on your grocery list.

• • • • • • • • • • • • • • • • • • • • • • • • • •

**Group items that are alike.** If you're running errands, group items you need to purchase by type of store—pharmacy, food, pet, hardware. Create your grocery list in categories like fresh fruits and vegetables, dairy products, meats and frozen foods.

• • • • • • • • • • • • • • • • • • • • • • • •

**Use acronyms.** No paper handy to write down things you need to remember? Try this: Create a word from the first letter of each item on your list. For example, C-R-O-W might mean "Call for theater tickets, Return library books, Order birthday cake, Water plants."

• • • • • • • • • • • • • • • • • • • • • • • •

**Use the first letter of each item** to create a funny phrase. To remember items you tend to forget in the morning rush (e.g., wallet, sunglasses, outgoing mail, lunch, hat), create the phrase "What smart, outrageous man laughs heartily." As you leave the house, silently repeat this phrase to make sure you have everything.

• • • • • • • • • • • • • • • • • • • • • • • •

**Create a rhyme**. If you frequently forget which way to turn a light bulb, say "righty-tighty, lefty-loosey." For treating shock, "If the face is red, raise the head; if the face is pale, raise the tail."

• • • • • • • • • • • • • • • • • • • • • • • •

**Think of your A, B, Cs.** When something slips your mind, try to recall the first letter of what you want to remember. Once you get the first letter, think of everything you can that starts with that letter and eventually you'll find the right word. If you don't remember within a half-dozen tries, move on. If it's something important, you'll probably remember it spontaneously later.

## Remembering names

**Use repetition.** Try to use a person's name two or three times during a conversation. It'll help you remember the name.

• • • • • • • • • • • • • • • • • • • • • • • • •

**Spell names in your head.** If you have difficulty remembering names, try spelling them in your head. Associating faces with the spelling of names activates multiple memory pathways in your brain.

• • • • • • • • • • • • • • • • • • • • • • • • •

**Link names to a place or occupation.** It's easier to remember something if you link it to something else. When you meet new people, associate their names with their occupations or the group in which you met them (e.g., Skier Bob). Picture them in that place with a nametag to identify them.

• • • • • • • • • • • • • • • • • • • • • • • • •

## Create a mental picture of the person.

To remember someone's name, picture the person, what they do, where they live or other things you can remember. This may bring to mind a letter of the alphabet, which you can build on by going through all the names you can think of that begin with that letter until the correct one comes to mind.

• • • • • • • • • • • • • • • • • • • • • • • • •

**Use association or word pictures** to remember names. Here are some examples to help you remember names by associating them with pictures: "Shave" for "Dave," "Cave-in" for "Kevin," "Cross" for "Chris." It may take practice before you can do this automatically.

• • • • • • • • • • • • • • • • • • • • • • • • •

**Rhyme names.** A tip for remembering names: Try to rhyme the person's name with a color, group or something else that associates the person with the name (e.g., Mr. Green Gene, Redheaded Deb, Bike Mike). Use a word or memory key that will remind you not only of the person but also of something about that person.

• • • • • • • • • • • • • • • • • • • • • • • • •

**Review the names of attendees** before meetings, events and reunions, especially if you haven't seen people recently. If possible, obtain a guest list prior to the event. If you have pictures to go along with the names, all the better.

• • • • • • • • • • • • • • • • • • • • • • • • •

**Ask people to help you remember names.**
Some people find it easy to remember people's names. If you have difficulty, however, be honest and tell people when you meet them. Ask them to remind you of their name the next time you meet.

• • • • • • • • • • • • • • • • • • • • • • • • • • • •

**Use a sense of humor**. If you regularly have memory lapses, make up a humorous response for common situations, such as "I'm having a senior moment" or "I didn't recognize you—you changed your clothes." At your next office party or reunion, try wearing a button that says, "Nice to see you. I can't remember your name either."

# Remembering dates

**Associate information with a date** you already know. You might remember that you had your last tetanus shot right after 9/11. That was in 2001, so another is needed in 2011. You might remember things happening the day before Halloween, a week after your birthday, two days after the Fourth of July or a month before Christmas.

• • • • • • • • • • • • • • • • • • • • • • • • • • • •

**Create a rhyme or song.** Remember in grade school you learned, "In 1492 Columbus sailed the ocean blue." Add new words to familiar tunes such as "Happy Birthday" or "Row, Row, Row Your Boat." Or be creative and write your own ditties.

• • • • • • • • • • • • • • • • • • • • • • • • • • • •

**Dates can become prices or a time.** For example, remember the year 1899 as $18.99 or February 14 as 2:14.

# Remembering numbers

**Keep a list of frequently dialed numbers** by the telephone. Type one list of phone numbers of people you call frequently and a second list of phone numbers of businesses, services and anyone you call long distance. Photocopy both lists, staple them back-to-back and slip them into a clear acetate sheet from an office supply store. For easy reference, keep a list at each phone in your home.

• • • • • • • • • • • • • • • • • • • • • • • • • • • • • •

**Saying numbers out loud** may help you remember addresses and phone numbers and even improve your ability to add and subtract numbers in your checkbook. If adding and subtracting numbers is a big problem, consider using a money-management computer software program that does the math for you.

• • • • • • • • • • • • • • • • • • • • • • • • • • • • • •

**Create words** to remember telephone numbers. Use the letters on the dial to create a word to help you remember. Commercial companies do this all the time (e.g., 1-800-verizon).

• • • • • • • • • • • • • • • • • • • • • • • • • • • • • •

**Look at the pattern you create** when you dial. Does it remind you of an X? Or an H? Some people find it easier to remember a pattern than a number.

• • • • • • • • • • • • • • • • • • • • • • • •

**Remember a telephone number** by creating a little melody that can be sung as you recite the number. Simultaneously using the left side of your brain (numbers) and the right side (melody) is a powerful memory aid.

• • • • • • • • • • • • • • • • • • • • • • • •

**Keep a calculator next to the phone** to quickly "write down" the number. You can enter the number more quickly on a keypad than you can write it down.

• • • • • • • • • • • • • • • • • • • • • • • •

**Purchase a cell phone with features** to help you remember. Some cell phones offer voice activated dialing. After you record the names and numbers of people you call regularly, simply push a button and speak the prerecorded name to dial the connection. Some cell phones allow you to record a short message or write a short note using the number and letter pad. Some have an alarm you can set. Shop for the cell phone with the features most helpful to you.

• • • • • • • • • • • • • • • • • • • • • • • •

# Using the telephone

**Get free directory assistance.** If you have a medical condition and a doctor verifies that you have trouble using a telephone book or remembering a phone number long enough to dial it, you may qualify for free directory assistance. Contact your telephone company's special needs or services department for more information.

• • • • • • • • • • • • • • • • • • • • • • • • • • • •

**Take note of automatic telephone** menu choices. If you call a clinic, pharmacy, store or business regularly that has a menu of options (Press 1 for hours, 2 for appointments, etc.), make note of the choices that connect you to the information, person or office you want to reach. Write them in your phone book so the next time you call you can enter the number without having to listen to every option.

• • • • • • • • • • • • • • • • • • • • • • • • • • • •

**Use a cordless phone** with a locator button. If you like the convenience of a cordless phone but keep misplacing the handset, purchase a phone with a locator button. When activated, this feature emits a loud beeping sound to help you find the handset between sofa cushions or in another room, wherever it may have been left.

• • • • • • • • • • • • • • • • • • • • • • • • • • • •

**The Amplified Photo Phone** may help keep you in touch with loved ones. Program each of the nine quick-dial buttons on the phone and add photos as visual cues of who will be called (mother, child, friend, doctor, emergency, etc.) when that button is pushed. To call, push the button with the appropriate picture. The phone also has a loud ringer helpful to people who are hard of hearing. About $50. Dynamic Living, 428 Hayden Station Road, Windsor, CT 06095-1302; 888-940-0605; www.dynamic-living.com.

**Put a red dot on your phone's "0" button** or the "0" on the dial so that older adults who may be unable to dial 911 will know which number to use to call in case of emergency.

**Put an address and phone label** on your phone for emergencies. Using a label maker or self-adhesive label, print your address and phone number and put a label on each telephone in your home. If you or a visitor needs to summon help, the necessary information will be right at your fingertips.

**Purchase a Telephone Hanger-Upper.** If a family member tends to leave the phone off the hook, the Automatic Telephone Hanger-Upper may be a solution. This device disconnects the phone line if the person forgets to place the handset back into the cradle. When another call comes in, the phone will ring even if the handset isn't in the cradle. Plugs into a wall outlet (adapter included). Telephone not included. Size: 3" x 4" x 1⅛". Ageless Design, Inc., 12633 159th Court North, Jupiter, FL 33478-6669; 800-752-3238; 561-745-0210; fax: 561-744-9572; email: cs@alzstore.com; www.alzstore.com.

## Finding things

**If you lose something,** breathe slowly and avoid panicking. If your brain is overtaxed and stressed, it will have difficulty remembering anything, so take a deep breath and count to 10. As you calm down, you should notice your thinking getting clearer.

• • • • • • • • • • • • • • • • • • • • • • • • •

**If you forget what you're doing** or lose something, stop and walk backward in your mind. Tell yourself to relax, close your eyes and retrace your steps mentally until you remember. If that doesn't work, physically retrace your route and go to where you last remember seeing the item you're looking for.

• • • • • • • • • • • • • • • • • • • • • • • •

**Put your car keys** with items you might forget. If you tend to leave coats, umbrellas or even groceries at a friend's house, put your car keys with the item you're likely to forget, such as in your coat pocket, on your umbrella handle or in your grocery bag. You can't go very far without remembering.

• • • • • • • • • • • • • • • • • • • • • • • •

**Keep a small container** filled with essentials (a little money, a pair of earrings, a spare tie) in your car's glove compartment.

• • • • • • • • • • • • • • • • • • • • • • • •

**Mark possessions you tend to lose.** Put your name and telephone number or address on umbrellas, books and other items you tend to leave behind. This will enable others to return them. *Note:* It's not a wise idea to put your address on your keys.

• • • • • • • • • • • • • • • • • • • • • • • •

# Using sticky notes

**When you're working on a task** and think of something unrelated, write down the thought on a sticky note and put it on your desk, door or mirror. When you're finished with your project, you can attend to the task on the note.

• • • • • • • • • • • • • • • • • • • • • • • • • • • • •

**Use sticky notes to indicate** future action needed. If you have a big pile of mail or work you need to sort, prioritize and act upon, use sticky notes to remind you of the action needed for each item in the pile. When you get to each item, you'll know what you have to do.

• • • • • • • • • • • • • • • • • • • • • • • • • • • • •

**Use sticky notes for errand reminders.** Sticky notes are a great invention because they have so many uses. Keep a pack in the car (with a pencil) and write notes to help you remember errands, appointments and schedules. Stick notes on the dashboard so what you need to remember is "in your face."

• • • • • • • • • • • • • • • • • • • • • • • • • • • • •

**Use bright sticky notes** to catch your eye. When you have a stack of things to do, indicate those that need special or immediate attention by using bright colored paper or a sticky note placed to catch your eye. You'll be less likely to overlook these things.

**Keep a sticky note** with your personal data assistant (PDA) so if you can't enter information right away (in the car, in poor lighting or when you're in a hurry), you'll have a place to write the note before entering it. Some PDAs come with a case that holds notes.

**Sticky notes can be used in dozens of ways** to help you remember. When scheduled to go to an event where you might want to take pictures, put a reminder note on the back of the door so you don't forget to take your camera. Put notes on the door before leaving town to remember to set the thermostat back, take out the garbage and make sure all appliances are turned off. If you have an appointment, put a note on the bedroom or bathroom mirror. To remember to make a long distance call after 5:00, put a note on the TV screen so you'll see it when you watch the news. Sticky notes on your refrigerator door will keep your grocery list handy.

# Making lists

**Shop with a list.** When you shop, whether for groceries, clothes, gifts or household items, always bring a list and keep a pencil with you. Cross out each item as you put it into the basket or purchase it.

. . . . . . . . . . . . . . . . . . . . . . . . . . . .

**Keep a list** of commonly used phone numbers by the telephone.

. . . . . . . . . . . . . . . . . . . . . . . . . . . .

**Keep a list of current doctors** and medications in your wallet.

. . . . . . . . . . . . . . . . . . . . . . . . . . . .

**Create a list of questions** to ask your doctor the next time you have an appointment.

. . . . . . . . . . . . . . . . . . . . . . . . . . . .

**Makes lists of anything you refer to** over and over again, from access numbers and passwords to things to pack in your suitcase when you travel.

. . . . . . . . . . . . . . . . . . . . . . . . . . . .

**Create a permanent packing list** to help you remember what to pack in your suitcase.

. . . . . . . . . . . . . . . . . . . . . . . . . . . .

**Make a sticky note list.** Write the things you need to do and want to remember on sticky notes. Put them on a notebook page or full size sheet of paper clipped to a clipboard or heavy sheet of cardboard (e.g., the cardboard on the back of a legal pad). Once you've completed the task, lift off the note and toss it out. It's quick and easy and you don't ever have to rewrite a list! You can also use scratch paper and tape instead of sticky notes.

## High tech and low tech aids

### Set an alarm to remind you to do tasks.
To keep track of tasks you need to do during the day (run errands, start dinner, take medications, etc.), set an alarm clock and carry it around with you (for alternative alarm devices, see Chapter 6: Medically Speaking). To help you remember what the alarm is reminding you to do, write the list of tasks and times on a white board (write on/wipe off) and post in a prominent and convenient place, such as the kitchen. As a double check to make sure you haven't forgotten anything, mark off each task as you do it.

• • • • • • • • • • • • • • • • • • • • • • • • •

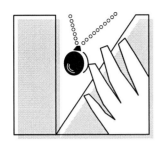

**Vibrating locket reminds you discreetly.** The Chronostone Personal Timer™ locket is an attractive aid for reminding women to take medication on time. Set the alarm and the locket silently vibrates at the same time each day. Includes a "second chance alarm." Easy Street Co., 384 Wickham Road, North Kingstown, R.I. 02852; 800-959-EASY; 800-959-3279; www.easystreetco.com.

• • • • • • • • • • • • • • • • • • • • • • • • •

**Program your pager with reminders** such as when to take your medications, move the sprinkler in the yard or perform other household tasks.

• • • • • • • • • • • • • • • • • • • • • • • • •

**Program numbers into your cell phone** if you have trouble remembering. The new models will store up to 100 phone numbers. Use speed-dial for important family numbers, so you can dial a number automatically by holding down only a single button.

• • • • • • • • • • • • • • • • • • • • • • • • •

**Personal data assistant.** If you like gadgets, purchase an electronic pocket organizer or personal data assistant (PDA) such as Palm Pilot. Use it to keep your address book, appointment calendar, notes and to-do lists. Some PDAs have a built-in tape recorder.

• • • • • • • • • • • • • • • • • • • • • • • • •

**Tape record reminders on audiocassette** and microcassette recorders and cell phones. Daily tasks, comforting messages and recipes can be put on the tapes. Pictures on the plastic cassette case and a magnifying glass could also be helpful.

**Record step-by-step instructions** on a StepPAD. "Play" repeats the cue as often as needed; "Forward" moves to the next step; "Rewind" goes back to the previous one. You can reprogram the StepPad easily, changing one step without affecting others in the sequence. Total of 72 seconds recording time. Batteries and clip included. Size: 2¼" x 3½" x ½". About $29. Attainment Company, Inc., PO Box 930160, Verona, WI 53593-0160; 800-327-4269; www.attainmentcompany.com.

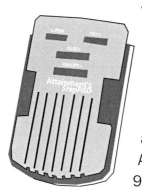

**Use an answering machine** to remember. When you are out and about and it isn't possible to write yourself a reminder note, use your cell phone to leave a message on your home answering machine.

**Take digital pictures** of class or meeting notes. If you have difficulty taking notes or remembering points at meetings or in class, take a digital picture of the noteboard or charts and import it into your computer to review later.

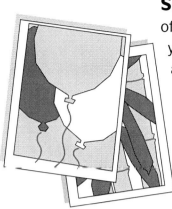

**Send a greeting card or postcard** with the help of the US Postal Service's NetPost CardStore. Are you notorious for forgetting your friend's birthday or anniversary? Spend an hour online at the CardStore and you can be sure that your card will be in the mailbox on time from now on. Choose from a collection of cards and pick the date to arrive, up to one year in advance. $2–3.50 per card includes postage. Check at your local post office or www.usps.com/netpost for details.

## Computers

**Use your home computer** to help remember where things are located. Create a document in your word processing program called WHERE.IT.IS. List the location of important papers and unusual items. To keep the document confidential, protect it with a password.

• • • • • • • • • • • • • • • • • • • • • • • •

**Set the alarm on your computer** to remind you to take a break and put your feet up, take your medication or attend to food cooking on the stove.

• • • • • • • • • • • • • • • • • • • • • • • •

**If you use email regularly,** send yourself reminder messages. An email message reduces clutter and doesn't get lost like scraps of paper might. You may be able to send the message days or weeks in advance to arrive on just the right day.

• • • • • • • • • • • • • • • • • • • • • • • •

**Write down access codes** or passwords backwards on a card in your wallet so no one else knows what they are.

• • • • • • • • • • • • • • • • • • • • • • • • • •

**Keep passwords in a dummy folder.** To keep track of computer and other passwords, write them on the inside cover of a dummy file folder. Remember what you called your dummy file by writing a clue (e.g., Grandmother's maiden name) on the bottom of your mouse pad or keyboard. You might want to write it backwards for added security.

• • • • • • • • • • • • • • • • • • • • • • • • • •

**Use one access code** or password for everything. If you have trouble remembering many different access codes for telephone lines, ATM pins and so forth, use the same access code for all, adding a suffix specific for each account (e.g., 2341MC for Mastercard) for added protection. For security sake, be very sure you keep your code number a secret.

• • • • • • • • • • • • • • • • • • • • • • • • • •

**Keep computer glasses at the computer.**
If you need glasses to work at the computer and they tend to wander off, cut a 1" piece of hook and loop fastener tape and stick it to the side of your computer monitor. Cut an opposing piece of fastener tape, 2" long, and fold it over a key ring. Attach the key ring to the fastener tape on the side of your monitor. Just insert the earpiece through the key ring and you will always know where your computer glasses are.

• • • • • • • • • • • • • • • • • • • • • • • • • •

**Use the AutoCorrect feature** on your computer. If you repeatedly have difficulty spelling a complicated word or name, take a few moments to program your fingers by typing the word or name ten times in a row. If this technique doesn't imprint the word on your mind, automatic features in your word processor will help you remember complicated words, names and phrases. In Microsoft Word, review the instructions for AutoCorrect and AutoText, both of which recall a word or phrase when you type a few letters. AutoCorrect operates with programmed shortcuts you create; AutoText recognizes the pattern of letters and automatically suggests the rest. See your computer Help feature for details.

• • • • • • • • • • • • • • • • • • • • • • •

**Use the Bookmark feature.** If you're working on a lengthy document and have to quit in the middle, create an electronic bookmark where you stopped so you can remember your place when you come back to it again. See your computer Help feature for details.

• • • • • • • • • • • • • • • • • • • • • • •

**Google it.** The next time you have trouble remembering something, try looking it up online. Even while you are talking on the phone, you can quickly search the Internet, find the information you need and avoid appearing unprepared. Google is a very discreet crutch for an ailing memory.

• • • • • • • • • • • • • • • • • • • • • • •

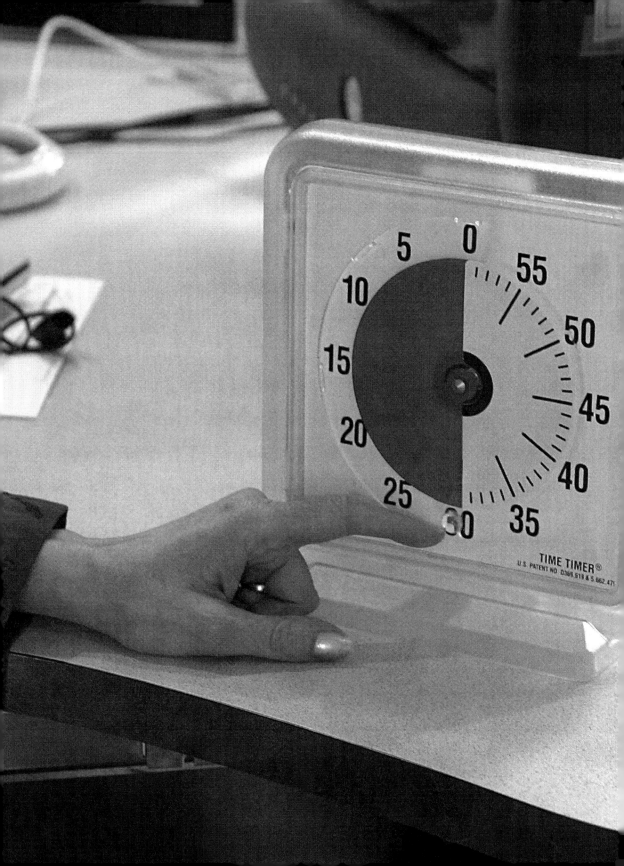

# 4

# a matter of time

"I wish I had better ways of keeping track of time, appointments, due dates and schedules." Sound familiar? If you're like me, you're like "mission control," in charge of running the home and family life. I know I must have specific ways of recording information, coordinating schedules and posting reminders so I don't forget, confuse or completely blow important events, checkups, deadlines and due dates. Perhaps the tips in this chapter will help you keep on top of things in a timely manner.

# ASSESSING YOUR NEEDS

**To help keep track of time, it would be helpful to:**

○ Count the seconds

○ Purchase a specialty watch or one with multiple features (day, date, alarm, etc.)

○ Use a pen that displays the day and date

○ Purchase a digital clock with large numbers

○ Create a daily clock with colorful pictures to highlight activities

○ Use a calendar to display events and activities

**To remember appointments, it would be helpful to:**

○ Use an erasable calendar

○ Post reminders on a do-it-yourself chalkboard

**To keep track of schedules, it would be helpful to:**

○ Use an appointment book as a personal scheduler

○ Use a notebook to track daily schedules

○ Use spiral index cards

○ Hang a large wall calendar with everyone's schedule visible

**To remember dates and deadlines, it would be helpful to:**

○ Write special events on a calendar in red ink

○ Use a pocket calendar to keep track of birthdays

○ Create a system for paying bills on time

○ Usc a pcrpctual calcndar to keep track of annual events

○ Use a TimePAD to get personalized reminders

**To provide support, it would be helpful to:**

○ Write down a set of sequenced instructions

# Telling time

**Count seconds** by saying 1001, 1002 and so forth. Need to time ten seconds? Sing the song "Happy Birthday" once.

**Purchase a stainless steel watch.** If you often forget to take off your watch when you hop in the shower, take a swim or participate in activities that might damage a traditional watch, consider a Freestyle Bump watch. It's scratch resistant, completely waterproof and sophisticated enough to wear to a formal dinner. About $60. Contact Freestyle USA for a dealer near you. 800-949-1563; www.freestyleusa.com.

**A watch that has a day and date feature** can help you remember the day of the week when no calendar is available.

**Purchase a pen** with a date and time feature if you don't wear a watch.

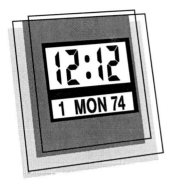

**A digital wall clock with large bold numbers** will help you keep track of the day, date and time. Available in a variety of styles from traditional to contemporary. About $25. Partshelf.com, 10138 S. Bode St. Unit C, Plainfield, IL 60544; 630-922-3659; www.giftngadget.com/wallclocks.

**Create a large, daily clock** to keep track of activities. Keep everyone informed of the daily schedule (breakfast, nap, exercise, visiting, etc.) by making a colorful wall clock with big bright numbers representing the hours of the day, and colorful pictures and words denoting the daily routine. Everyone will know at a glance "what time it is!"

**To help with time and sequencing,** create a calendar for the month with large squares (2" x 2") and draw little pictures in the squares to identify upcoming events. Draw a birthday cake with candles to signify a birthday party; books to signify a trip to the library; a bunny, jack-o'-lantern, heart or shamrock to signify special holiday celebrations. Each day, using a dark crayon or marker, cross out the previous day on the calendar.

# Remembering appointments

**Keep track of your family's appointments** with an erasable calendar you design to meet your specific needs. Start with a blank calendar page with six rows of seven boxes. Fill in the days of the week in the first row but leave the name of the month and the dates blank. Make your calendar whatever size works for you—small enough to fit where you want to put it but large enough to record all the information you need. Take two—one for this month and one for the next— to your printer or copy shop and have them laminated. Using dry erase markers (regular markers will cause permanent stains), write the month and each day's date in the appropriate boxes. You can use this same technique to create a custom message board for a to-do list, medicine schedule or TV guide.

• • • • • • • • • • • • • • • • • • • • • • • • • • •

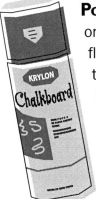

**Post reminders and appointments** on a do-it-yourself chalkboard. Almost any flat surface (doors, cabinets, etc.) can be turned into a chalkboard by spraying Krylon Chalkboard Paint on it. Available in green or black. $5–7 per can. Check www.krylon.com for store locations.

• • • • • • • • • • • • • • • • • • • • • • • •

# Keeping track of schedules

**Use an appointment book** to keep track of your personal schedule. Purchase an appointment book with a calendar in the format that works best for you (day, week or month at a glance) and a place to write, organized into sections like Things to Do, Calls to Make, Errands and Groceries. Create a section in the front or back of the calendar where you can write frequently used phone numbers. (If there isn't a blank page for the telephone numbers, glue a piece of paper over a page of writing or a picture you don't need.) When creating your phone number page, group the numbers in categories: Doctors and medical clinics, friends, long distance contacts, local businesses. Also write down the directions and codes for retrieving your messages from your answering machine.

• • • • • • • • • • • • • • • • • • • • • • •

**Track daily schedules,** events, medical symptoms and so forth in a notebook. Use a spiral notebook (if left handed, a steno book may work better) and start a new page each day. Record the time of day and what happened, for example:

8:00 Breakfast—French toast
9:00 Talked to sister Ann

Include appointments, activities, thoughts and things of interest in your book.

• • • • • • • • • • • • • • • • • • • • • • •

**To remember what needs to be done,**
purchase a spiral book of index cards. Write the date
at the top of each card (one day per card). Then list
the day's schedule and the specific time, if applicable.
As each item on the list is completed, cross it out.
At the end of the day, tear out the card and discard
it, or if you want a record of activities, file the card
chronologically in an index file box.

• • • • • • • • • • • • • • • • • • • • • • • • • •

**Hang a wall calendar with large squares** in
a prominent location to keep track of everyone's
schedule. Assign each family member a different ink
color and let everyone record their activities on the
calendar using their assigned colored pen. You'll know
at a glance who needs to be where at what time.

# Recording dates and deadlines

**Mark the date of birthdays** and anniversaries
on a calendar in red ink so it's easy to see. Write the
person's telephone number next to the name so you
don't forget anyone's special day.

• • • • • • • • • • • • • • • • • • • • • • • • • •

**Keep track of birthdays** and other important dates in a pocket calendar. Begin each year with a new pocket calendar, the kind that has a square for each day, and write in upcoming events, celebrations and birthdays. Take the calendar with you to the card store and purchase cards for the entire year. Keep the calendar and cards in a folder or binder with 12 pockets, one for each month. At the beginning of the month, address the cards, marking the date to mail in the spot where the stamp goes. When the date arrives, apply a stamp over the date and mail.

• • • • • • • • • • • • • • • • • • • • • • • • • • •

**Create a system to pay bills on time.** When the mail comes, open all the bills at once and write the due dates on a big kitchen calendar. Every day, perhaps in the morning or after dinner when you have your coffee, check the calendar and send out any bill with a due date approaching. Once this becomes routine, you'll always be on top of your bills and need never pay another late fee.

• • • • • • • • • • • • • • • • • • • • • • • • • • •

**Keep track of annual events** with a perpetual calendar. Purchase a calendar with dates only (no year or days of the week) and keep track of birthdays and anniversaries without having to transfer them to a new calendar each year. As long as you remember to turn the page each day, this kind of calendar will make it easy to remember important dates year after year.

• • • • • • • • • • • • • • • • • • • • • • • • • •

**Use a TimePAD** to signal when to leave for appointments, begin tasks or take medications. This device automatically plays back up to five personalized reminders (e.g., "It's 8:30—take your medication"). Records up to 72 seconds of speech divided among five messages. Also functions as an expressive communication aid. Users simply press the message buttons to talk. Batteries and clip included. Size: $2^1/_8$" x $3^7/_8$" x $3/_8$". About $29. Attainment Company, Inc., PO Box 930160, Verona, WI 53593-0160; 800-327-4269; www.attainmentcompany.com.

• • • • • • • • • • • • • • • • • • • • • •

# Providing support

wet the toothbrush

ply toothpaste

brush teeth

**Create a set of sequenced instructions.** To help someone with memory difficulties remember how to do tasks such as make a meal, brush teeth or get dressed, take pictures of each step in the process. Number the instructions and post them on a wall, in a photo sleeve or album, or on a key ring near where the activity will take place. For a preprinted set of cards relating to various activities, contact Attainment Company, Inc., PO Box 930160, Verona, WI 53593-0160; 800-327-4269; www.attainmentcompany.com.

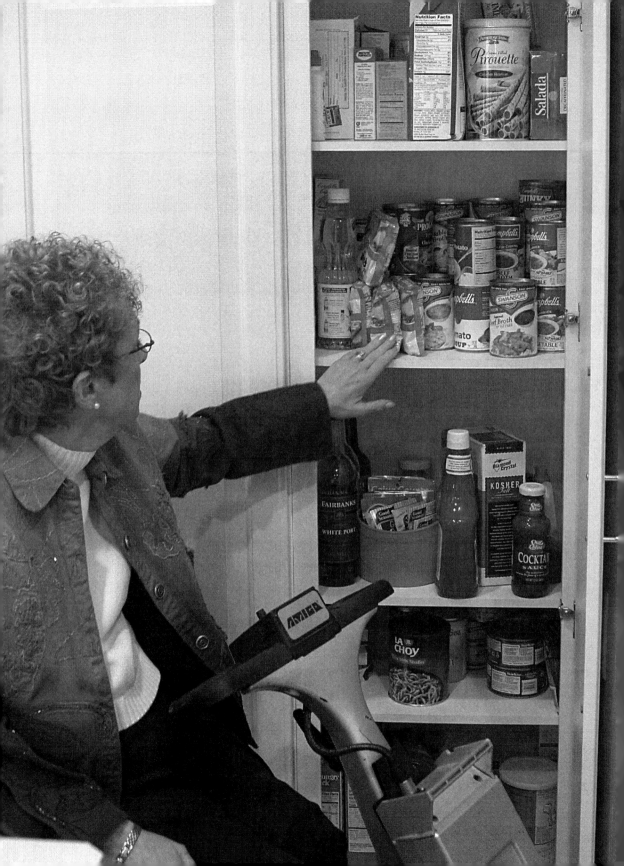

# 5

# your house and home

My husband and I were fortunate to live in a home that could easily be adapted to my increasing needs. We needed to make the home accessible to my wheelchair and also to create an environment that would allow my helpers and me to know where things went, how they were organized and why. Whether buying an appliance, doing mundane chores or using unique products to help me remain independent, I wanted to reduce stress and keep on top of the things I needed to manage around my house. In this chapter you'll find techniques to use around your house that will reduce the number of things you have to remember and remove some of the stress in your life.

# ASSESSING YOUR NEEDS

**To find stored items, it would be helpful to:**

○ Label the contents of cabinets and drawers

○ Put pictures of contents on outside of drawers and cabinet doors

○ Use drawer organizers in contrasting colors

○ Use a flashlight to find things in cupboards

○ Use transparent containers to see what's inside

**To use appliances safely, it would be helpful to:**

○ Purchase products that automatically shut off

○ Buy a stove with removable buttons

○ Identify electric cords with color-coded ties

○ Wrap appliance cords in cardboard tubes

**To navigate in the home more easily, it would be helpful to:**

○ Decorate bedroom and bathroom doors

○ Use luminous paint or reflector tape to show the way

○ Use a MotionPAD™ to signal a door opening

○ Decorate sliding glass doors for safety

**To use keys more easily, it would be helpful to:**

- ○ Wear my house key around my neck
- ○ Keep extra keys in my wallet
- ○ Mark my house key with fluorescent tape
- ○ Replace self-locking locks with key locks
- ○ Hide a set of house keys
- ○ Purchase a beeping key chain
- ○ Use a remote control key locator

**To use faucets more easily, it would be helpful to:**

- ○ Purchase an EZ Flo automatic water wand
- ○ Use a touchless faucet
- ○ Label the hot water faucet

**To use lights and thermostats more easily, it would be helpful to:**

- ○ Install a nightlight in the bathroom
- ○ Install a motion detector
- ○ Put new lightbulbs in outdoor fixtures before winter
- ○ Use a setback thermostat

# ASSESSING YOUR NEEDS

**To remember in the kitchen, it would be helpful to:**

○ Group frozen foods together

○ Use a portable timer

○ Use a timer that must be turned off

○ Arrange spices in alphabetical order

○ Purchase a photo cookbook

○ Give away copies of recipes instead of originals

○ Keep recipes in small photo albums

○ Make grocery lists with box tops and labels

○ Use placemats with tableware outlines

○ Lock the dishwasher door to indicate clean dishes

**To remember in the bathroom, laundry and bedroom, it would be helpful to:**

○ Replace toothbrushes with each change in season

○ Post laundry care instructions near the washer and dryer

○ Keep a list of stain removal tips

○ Tie a knot in clothing to indicate a stain

○ Purchase different colors for different sized sheets

○ Use a slipper to remember to do something

○ Keep morning and bedtime medication at the bedside

○ Use a weekly pill organizer

**To remember outside the house, it would be helpful to:**

- ○ Construct a circular path to making walking safer
- ○ Decorate in a distinctive way
- ○ Remind visitors not to block the mailbox
- ○ Wear a reminder bracelet
- ○ Paint tool handles with fluorescent paint
- ○ Use self-watering pots

**To be safe at home, it would be helpful to:**

- ○ Label every circuit breaker
- ○ Change alarm batteries every year
- ○ Separate items that might cause confusion
- ○ Register a loved one with the Safe Return Program
- ○ Protect property with Codetag™ Property Recover services
- ○ Remember to bring in the mail with an electronic mailbox chime
- ○ Avert disaster with a flooding alarm

## Maintaining consistency

**If you're helping someone in the home,** resist the temptation to move things or reorganize. Maintain consistency by leaving things in their familiar places.

## Cabinets, drawers and storage

**Label the contents of each cabinet** and drawer, including file cabinets, linen cabinets and dresser drawers. Label shelves, dividers, boxes and containers so everyone knows what goes where. This is especially helpful when company comes or you're sick and someone is helping you. If everything is labeled, they don't have to keep asking you where things go.

• • • • • • • • • • • • • • • • • • • • • • • • •

**Use pictures on kitchen drawers** and cabinet doors to help someone find things like silverware, plates, napkins and cups. A picture of a box of breakfast cereal, for example, could go where cereals are kept.

• • • • • • • • • • • • • • • • • • • • • •

**Drawer organizers in contrasting colors** will help you remember where specific items are stored. For example: All red-topped containers go under the sink and all blue-topped containers go back to the workbench. Organizers can be found at discount, kitchen or grocery stores.

• • • • • • • • • • • • • • • • • • • • • • • •

**Keep a small flashlight handy** for those times you can't remember what's "back there" in deep cupboards and cabinets.

• • • • • • • • • • • • • • • • • • • • • • • •

**Use transparent plastic containers** to see what's inside. Write the contents of the container on an index card and place it where you can see it when you open the drawer or door. Even if your memory is good, this will help you locate items quickly.

## Appliances and electronics

**Purchase products** with an automatic shutoff feature. Many of the newer coffeemakers, irons, clock radios, copiers, printers, curling irons and computers automatically shut off after a certain amount of time has lapsed.

• • • • • • • • • • • • • • • • • • • • • • • •

**Purchase a stove** with removable buttons or dials as a safety measure for people who may forget the stove is on. It is also helpful if the controls are along the front of the appliance, so the person cooking doesn't have to reach across the burners to turn the stove on and off.

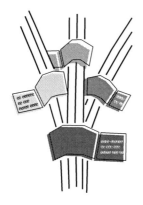

**Identify electric cords** with color-coded cable ties. If you have a tangle of electric cords in the kitchen, computer room or entertainment center, straighten up the mess by securing the cords with cable ties, readily available at hardware, electronics or office supply stores. Use a different color for each appliance to make it easier to find a specific cord.

**Wrap individual appliance cords** in cardboard tubes. Know at a glance which cord goes with which appliance by winding up the cord and sliding it into an empty toilet paper or paper towel tube. To make it easy to match the right cord with the right appliance, write the name of the appliance on the tube and keep it in a kitchen drawer or inside the appliance.

# Doors and doorways

**Decorate the door** to make a room easier to find. If a hallway full of similar doors makes it difficult to find your way, make important doorways, like those to the bedroom and bathroom easier to find by painting or decorating the door in a distinctive way.

• • • • • • • • • • • • • • • • • • • • • • • • •

**Use luminous paint or reflector tape** to show the way. If a family member gets out of bed in the middle of the night and becomes confused finding the way, paint the door frames of the bedroom and bathroom with luminous paint to help the person find the way in the dark. Or create a path with reflector tape leading from the bedroom to the bathroom.

• • • • • • • • • • • • • • • • • • • • • • • Ⓐ🖐

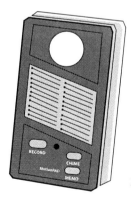

**MotionPAD™ alerts you** to a door opening. Placed near or on a door, this motion sensitive device chimes or plays a single prerecorded message when the door is opened. Messages are easily recorded and can be locked to prevent re-recording. Uses four AA batteries. About $39. Attainment Company, PO Box 930160, Verona, WI 53593-0160; 800-327-4269; fax: 800-942-3865; www.AttainmentCompany.com.

• • • • • • • • • • • • • • • • • • • • • Ⓐ🖐

**Put decorative decals or pictures** on sliding glass doors to alert you that the door is closed and to prevent you from walking into it.

## Locks and keys

**Put your house key on a string** or shoelace that you wear around your neck. Make it a habit to put the necklace on first thing in the morning and you'll never accidentally lock yourself out of the house.

• • • • • • • • • • • • • • • • • • • • • • • • • •

**Keep an extra house and car key** in your wallet.

• • • • • • • • • • • • • • • • • • • • • • • • • •

**Put a piece of fluorescent tape** on either side of your house key lock and on your keys to make it easier to find the lock and the right key in the dark.

• • • • • • • • • • • • • • • • • • • • • • • • • •

**Change the locks on your exterior doors** from self-locking to those that must be locked with a key. This will keep you from inadvertently locking yourself out of the house.

• • • • • • • • • • • • • • • • • • • • • • • • • •

**Keep a hidden set of house keys.** For those times when you inadvertently lock yourself out of the house, keep an extra set of keys in a hidden location that's easy for you to remember but difficult for a potential burglar to find.

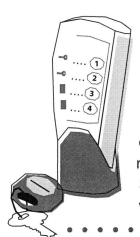

**Beeping key chain.** If you often find yourself searching for your keys, attach them to a beeping key chain and summon them easily by whistling or clapping your hands. Be aware that this key chain may also beep when any whistle-like sound is made. If that would be problematic, choose a place for your keys and always keep them in this spot. About $7. From ElderCorner; 877-883-5337; www.eldercorner.com.

**Use a remote control key locator** to keep track of your keys, PDA, wallet and cellphone. Attach color-coded receivers to items you tend to misplace. When you can't find an item, press the matching color-coded pager on the wireless transmitter and the receiver will answer with a loud alarm. Transmits up to 60 feet, through floors, walls and even sofa cushions. Includes two color-coded key rings and two slim, color-coded receivers to attach to other items. About $60. From Brookstone; 800-846-3000; www.brookstone.com.

# Faucets

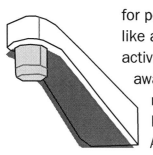

**EZ Flo automatic faucet control** turns water off automatically. This inexpensive device is designed for people who have trouble turning knobs. A stick-like attachment hooks onto your sink's faucet and is activated by a slight push. When you take your hand away, the water turns off. Knowing the water will never be left running will give you peace of mind. It works in the kitchen, bathroom or laundry. About $10 for one, $15 for two. International Environmental Solutions, Inc., 2830 Scherer Dr., Suite 310, St. Petersburg, Florida 33716; 800-972-8348; www.internationalenvironmentalsolutions.com.

**A touchless faucet has an electric eye** that senses a person's hands in front of it and turns the water on and off automatically. It can be preset to a specific temperature to avoid scalding. It may require professional installation. About $330–440. Contact a plumbing contractor or www.smarthome.com.

**Mark the hot water faucet** with red nail polish. If you have difficulty remembering which water faucet has hot water and which has cold, mark the hot water faucet with a dab of red polish.

# Lighting

**Install a nightlight in the bathroom** and leave the door open to make it easier to find your way in the night.

• • • • • • • • • • • • • • • • • • • • • • • • • •

**Install a motion detector** to switch on lights. If remembering to turn the lights off is a problem at your house, install a motion detector light switch that automatically turns the light on when you enter a room and turns it off when you leave. Some models come with adjustable timers with a maximum 20-minute delay. If you use a motion detector in the bedroom, you can safely get into bed before the light turns off. Lights can also be operated normally with a manual override feature. Readily available at hardware stores. About $25.

• • • • • • • • • • • • • • • • • • • • • • • • • •

**Putting new lightbulbs** in your outdoor light fixtures before winter arrives cuts down on the chances that you'll have to replace a bulb in bad weather. Remember to do this by replacing all the bulbs on the same day you turn back the clocks at the end of daylight savings time. You can use the old bulbs indoors or reinstall them outside in the spring.

• • • • • • • • • • • • • • • • • • • • • • • • • •

# Thermostats

**Use a setback thermostat** to regulate the temperature of your home automatically. For example, program the thermostat to drop to 65 degrees when you go to bed and rise to 72 degrees before you get out of bed. In summer, you can program your air conditioning in the same way. Some setback thermostats allow you to select different settings for weekdays and weekends, while others allow you to program each day individually. They're generally easy to install and can be purchased at hardware stores. If you want help selecting a thermostat for your needs or don't want to install it yourself, contact a heating or cooling contractor in your area. An electrician can also install these thermostats.

# The kitchen

**Group frozen foods together.** If you store food in a freezer for later use, whether leftovers or dishes cooked ahead for the holidays, group similar items together in one large plastic container. Use different colored covers for different groupings (vegetables, desserts, entrees, etc.) to find food quickly. Purchase containers at grocery and discount stores.

• • • • • • • • • • • • • • • • • • • • • • • • • • • • •

**Use a portable timer when cooking.** If you must leave the kitchen while cooking, take a portable timer with you. The ding will remind you that you have something on the stove or in the oven.

• • • • • • • • • • • • • • • • • • • • • • • • • • • •

**Use a timer or an alarm clock** that you have to turn off, as opposed to one that rings only once, to remind yourself to turn on the oven to start dinner.

• • • • • • • • • • • • • • • • • • • • • • • • • • • •

**Arrange your spices in alphabetical order** to make it easier to find them quickly and see when you need to purchase more.

• • • • • • • • • • • • • • • • • • • • • • • • • • • •

**Photo cookbook.** For those who want to cook but have difficulty reading, comprehending or following directions, *Home Cooking* offers 37 healthy, easy-to-prepare conventional and microwave recipes with step-by-step photo instructions. This vividly illustrated 160-page cookbook and instructor's guide is printed in color with laminated pages and is displayed in an easel binder for easy viewing. About $49. Attainment Company, Inc., 504 Commerce Parkway, PO Box 930160, Verona, WI 53593-0160; 800-327-4269; www.attainmentcompany.com.

• • • • • • • • • • • • • • • • • • • • • •

**Share copies of your recipes** with friends. If the original becomes unreadable or you lose it, your friends can give you the recipe.

• • • • • • • • • • • • • • • • • • • • • • • •

**Keep favorite recipes** in 4" x 6" photo albums. The plastic sleeves are perfect for organizing recipe cards as well as recipes torn out of magazines. They are compact enough to tuck in almost anywhere, so you might want to create one for salads, entrees, desserts, holidays and so forth. As an added bonus, you can wipe any spills off your recipes.

• • • • • • • • • • • • • • • • • • • • • • • •

**Use box tops and labels** to create grocery lists. To help you remember what to put on your grocery list, place box tops and labels of packaged food in a self-sealing bag attached to your refrigerator with a large magnet. When it's time to make your grocery list, add items from the bag. If others shop for you, they will have the size and brand of items you need.

• • • • • • • • • • • • • • • • • • • • • • • •

**To help you set the table correctly,** remember that "left" has four letters and so does "fork." "Right" has five letters, as do "knife" and "spoon."

• • • • • • • • • • • • • • • • • • • • • • • •

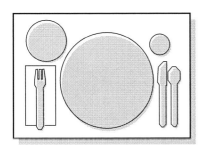

**Placemats with tableware outlines** make remembering how to set the table easy. Draw outlines of tableware (plate, bowl, tumbler, knife, fork and spoon) on paper placemats and laminate. To set the table, match the item to the outline. Or purchase a Table Setting, which includes four plastic tableware sets and four illustrated placemats. About $69. Attainment Company, Inc., PO Box 930160, Verona, WI 53593-0160; 800-327-4269; fax: 800-942-3865; www.AttainmentCompany.com.

**A locked dishwasher door** means dishes are clean. When you need to take a clean dish out of the dishwasher but do not have time to empty it, lock the door again so everyone will know the dishes inside are clean. Doing so will keep you from inadvertently putting dirty dishes in with the clean ones.

## The bathroom

**Replace your toothbrush** with each change of season. Dentists remind us to use a new toothbrush every three months. In January, buy four toothbrushes in colors that remind you of the changing seasons (e.g., white for winter, green for spring, yellow for summer, orange for autumn.) Throw out your old brush on the first day of spring, summer, fall and winter.

# Laundry

**Post laundry care instructions** near your washer and dryer. Tack an index card to a bulletin board or inside cabinet doors indicating how much and what kind of cleaning products to use, water levels and temperature settings. The note can also remind you of other special care instructions such as to keep Velcro™ fasteners closed so they don't collect lint or snag garments.

• • • • • • • • • • • • • • • • • • • • • • • • • •

**Keep a list of stain removal tips,** techniques and products in your laundry room to remind you how to treat specific problems.

• • • • • • • • • • • • • • • • • • • • • • • • • •

**Tie a knot in clothing** to remind you of a stain or repair that needs attention. After taking off a stained garment or one that needs repair, tie a knot in a sleeve or leg to remind you to pretreat or repair it before washing. Of course, if you take the time to pretreat a stain immediately, you won't have to remember.

• • • • • • • • • • • • • • • • • • • • • • • • • •

# The bedroom

**Purchase different colors and patterns** for different size sheets (twin, full, queen, king ) to help you identify the size of a sheet at a glance. For example, buy solid colors for queen size beds, flowers for full size beds, and geometric or cartoon designs for twin size beds.

• • • • • • • • • • • • • • • • • • • • • •

**Use your slipper to remember.** If you tend to think of things you need to do while trying to fall asleep, take one of your slippers from the floor next to the bed and toss it to another part of the room. When you wake up and can't find your slipper, you'll be more likely to remember the task that needs to be done.

• • • • • • • • • • • • • • • • • • • • • •

**Keep your morning medication** and a glass of water at your bedside so you remember to take it first thing in the morning. If your medication takes time to work, go back to sleep for a few minutes.

• • • • • • • • • • • • • • • • • • • • • •

**Put your bedtime pill on your nightstand** so you'll remember to take it right before bed. Keep extra pills and a straw in your nightstand, too.

• • • • • • • • • • • • • • • • • • •

**Use a weekly pill organizer** to keep track of doses. If you're worried you might not remember whether you took a pill, fill a weekly organizer with your pills and take each day's dose from the appropriate section.

# Outside the house

**A circular path can make walking** outside safer. Design a looped or circular path in your yard that will lead the walker back to the door. Provide prominent landmarks (a bench, brightly colored birdhouse, patch of flowers or decorative sculpture) along the way to make the walk interesting. Markers are especially important at the halfway point and near the door as points of reference.

**To find your way home more easily,** install a distinctive mailbox, paint your door a bright color, add large contrasting house numbers or decorate the entrance in a unique way. Not only will it be easier for you to find your home, but friends and emergency personnel will find it more easily.

**Don't block the mailbox.** If a car blocks your mailbox, the mail carrier won't deliver the mail. Remind visitors with a pleasant sign on your mailbox post.

**Use a bracelet to remind yourself** to turn off the hose. When watering the yard or garden, take an old bracelet and put it around your wrist to remind yourself that the water is on. When you're finished watering, take the bracelet off and put it around the faucet so it's ready to use the next time you turn on the water.

• • • • • • • • • • • • • • • • • • • • • •

**Paint garden tools with fluorescent paint** or wrap the handles with bright reflective tape. Not only will your tools be easier to find if you leave them out in the yard, but they will more likely come back to you when borrowed.

• • • • • • • • • • • • • • • • • • • • • •

**Replace traditional pots** with self-watering pots or planters, which come in a variety of styles and sizes. At the bottom of the pot is a slotted plastic inset with an easy-fill water reservoir, which is accessible from the outside of the pot. Plant as usual and water thoroughly from the top of the pot. After the soil is saturated, fill the water reservoir below. The soil acts as a wick, taking only the water it needs. Gardener's Supply Company; 800-427-3363; www.gardeners.com.

• • • • • • • • • • • • • • • • • • • • • •

# Household safety

**Label every circuit breaker.** To save time and energy identifying which circuit breaker switch will shut off the electricity to a specific part of your home, label every breaker switch. Here's an easy way to identify each breaker: Turn on a radio or TV with the volume loud enough to hear when you're at the circuit breaker box. When you flip the correct breaker, the radio or TV will shut off. Repeat this process for each room in the house, keeping in mind that laundry rooms and bathrooms may have more than one breaker. Kitchens may have separate breakers for major appliances, so you may want to check each outlet. In a very large home, enlist the aid of a friend to tell you via portable phone or walkie-talkie when the radio or TV goes off.

• • • • • • • • • • • • • • • • • • • • • • • • • •

**Change alarm batteries once a year.** A smoke alarm, radon detector or other battery-powered device is only as reliable as the batteries that operate it. To keep your family safe, be sure to change the batteries once a year. A good way to remember to change the batteries is to do so on the day of an annual event. For example, change the batteries at Thanksgiving as part of your holiday preparations. Or choose a birthday, anniversary or the end of daylight savings time in the fall. If you are unable to change the batteries yourself, contact your local fire department for assistance.

• • • • • • • • • • • • • • • • • • • • • • • • • •

**Separate items that may cause confusion**
and store them in different places. For example, don't leave shaving cream in a drawer next to the toothpaste. Remove stove and oven knobs when not in use, remove or lock up sharp knives, and put away kitchen appliances such as blenders and toasters.

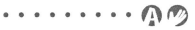

**Safe Return Program.** If you live with a confused adult, here are some suggestions for keeping the person safe: Place a pocket card with simple instructions, such as "call home" (with a phone number below), in your loved one's clothing or wallet. If that isn't practical, purchase a Safe Return bracelet (with the person's name, address and phone number on it) from the Alzheimer's Association and ask a doctor to place it on the person's wrist during an appointment. (It's likely to be better received from a doctor.) If the bracelet is placed on the individual's dominant hand, it will be more difficult to undo the clasp. Attach the bracelet to a belt loop or to shoelaces if the person is reluctant to wear it. For more information contact the Safe Return Program at 888-572-8566. Also try to determine the cause of wandering—it may simply be a signal that your loved one is looking for something, such as the bathroom, or is seeking a meaningful activity or reassurance. Some experts believe taking your loved one for a vigorous daily walk helps reduce wandering.

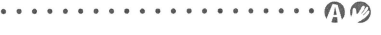

**Codetag™ Property Recovery Services** tracks and organizes the return of property if found after being lost or stolen. Their kit includes adhesive labels, iron-on clothing labels, key tags and luggage or bag tags—each with a unique serial number. You attach the labels to your personal items and register them with the company. If you lose a marked item and it's found, the finder is encouraged to contact the company to claim a reward provided by Codetag™. The company then arranges for the item's return, keeping your identity secure (shipping charges may apply). Subscription service is $9.95 for three years' protection; fee is waived if you purchase ID labels, starting at $1.95, from Codetag™. Codetag Property Recovery Systems, 369-B Third Street, Suite 121, San Rafael, CA 94901; 800-939-8247; www.codetag.com.

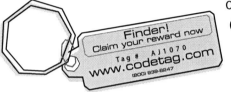

**An electronic mailbox chime alert** will remind you to bring in the mail. A wireless sensor attached to your mailbox alerts you to the arrival of the mail with an audible and visual signal in your home. In addition, transmitters may be attached to home and garage doors, providing added security by informing you whenever a door is opened. About $22–50. Available where home electronic and security equipment is sold and also from SmartHome, 16542 Millikan Ave., Irvine, CA 92606-5027; 800-762-7846; www. smarthome.com.

**Flooding alarms avert disaster.** Flooding alarms, designed for use in basements and laundry rooms to notify you if water is detected on the floor, are inexpensive insurance in the bathroom. The detector plugs into the wall (battery operated versions also available) with a sensor wire that leads to the floor. If the wire comes in contact with water (e.g., from an overflowing tub), the alarm lets you know. Great in the kitchen, laundry room or anywhere a water leak or overflow is possible. $10–15. Available at hardware stores or from SmartHome, 16542 Millikan Ave., Irvine, CA 92606-5027; 800-762-7846; www. smarthome.com.

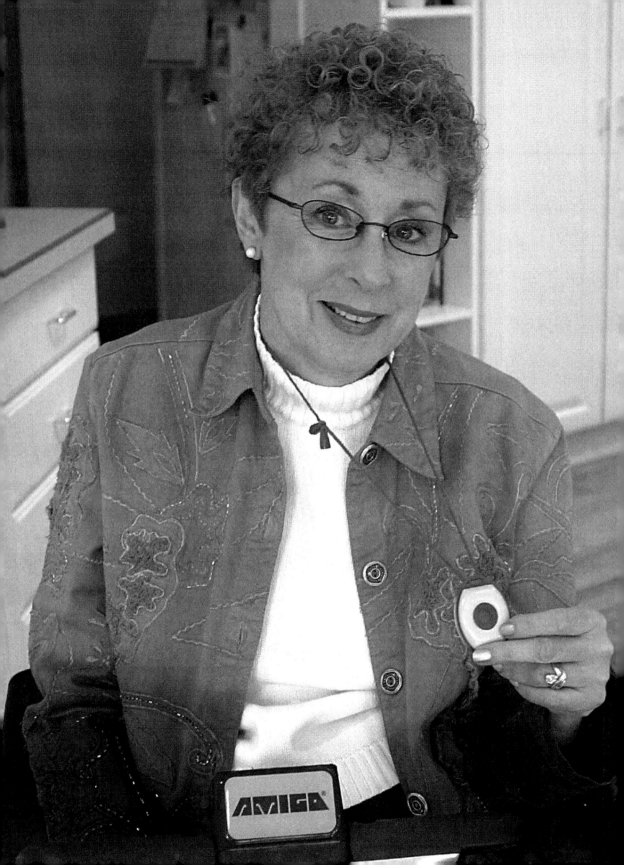

# 6

# medically speaking

When I was diagnosed with MS, I was overwhelmed with all the medically-related information I had to keep track of. Although it is quite common for people with MS to experience memory problems, I did not appear to have many of those issues. I did, however, feel like my mind was stretched to the limit with details of my medical history like what medications I was taking, why I was taking them, how long I had been taking them, their side effects and when to take them. Remembering appointments, what each doctor said and the purpose of medical treatments made me anxious. I realized I had to be the one in charge of my healthcare—no one was going to take care of me but ME. This chapter will help you manage the details of your health or the health of those you care for.

# ASSESSING YOUR NEEDS

**To understand and keep track of medical contact information, it would be helpful to:**

○ Write information on index cards

○ Create a personal health history

○ Wear a medical alert tag

○ Visit approved and respected medical websites

○ Contact well-respected organizations and research facilities

○ Keep a progress calendar

**To learn about medication, it would be helpful to:**

○ Ask for an explanation from the pharmacist

○ Learn medical abbreviations

○ Make sure medications are fresh

○ Write down why medication was prescribed

○ Set up automatic refills

○ Place a standing order

○ Keep extra medication on hand

○ Carry copies of prescriptions when traveling

○ Use a pharmacy with a national network

**CHAPTER 6** Medically Speaking

**To organize medications, it would be helpful to:**

○ Pre-package medications
○ Separate daily medication dose in the bottle
○ Use pill organizers
○ Use a Talking Rx™
○ Ask the pharmacist to prepackage pills

**To remember to take mediations, it would be helpful to:**

○ Create a schedule for taking meds
○ Post reminders on a bulletin board
○ Place medications in strategic locations
○ Keep meds handy in decorative containers
○ Use letter codes to remember when to take pills
○ Use time-release medications
○ Use drawings to identify injection sites
○ Use jewelry placement to remember to alternate injection sites
○ Mark syringes with a marking pen

**To use devices to remember to take mediations, it would be helpful to:**

○ Buy a MeDose™ reminder watch
○ Purchase a MedGlider™ System pillbox
○ Use a digital sports watch

# ASSESSING YOUR NEEDS

**To schedule appointments, it would be helpful to:**

○ Set up annual appointments around annual events

○ Mark the calendar as a reminder to set appointments

○ Write appointment dates down on business cards

○ Write the date temporarily on the palm of my hand

○ Ask for a reminder call

**To communicate with medical professionals, it would be helpful to:**

○ Be open and honest

○ Take a list of questions to appointments

○ Ask for videotape instructions for special procedures to repeat at home

○ Write instructions on self-adhesive labels

**To get support, it would be helpful to:**

○ Contact national health organizations

○ Use a national network of independent living centers

○ Seek assistance from social workers

○ Find resources at ElderCarelink

**To provide support, it would be helpful to:**

○ Keep a diary and communication notebook

○ Post instructions in a prominent place

○ Create step-by-step instructions

○ Remember the warning signs of stroke

# Medical information

**Keep important medical** and contact information on an index card. During medical emergencies it can be difficult to remember your name, not to mention your medications, doctors and emergency contact information. A simple way to keep important medical information handy is to use an index card. On one side of the card put the names and telephone numbers of your doctors, therapists, counselors, hospitals and clinics. You may also want to include the name of your clergyperson, family members or close friends. On the other side of the card, write the names of the medications you are taking, the dosage, time of day you take the drug, what the drug is for and how long you have been taking it. Don't forget to include any allergies you have to medications, preservatives and so forth. Keep the index card updated and near your driver's license in your wallet or purse so it's handy when you need it.

• • • • • • • • • • • • • • • • • • • • • • • • •

**Create a personal health history.** Remember important medical information by creating a binder where you keep a record of medical problems, medications, immunizations, allergies, dates of past hospitalizations and procedures, family medical history and more. Also keep copies of insurance information and legal documents such as Power of Attorney and Advance Medical Directives. A preprinted system, "Your Personal Health and Medical History," is divided into 10 categories (e.g., personal information, medications, hospitalizations, emergency contacts) with detailed, easy-to-fill-out medical information forms and legal documents. This invaluable resource comes in extremely handy in case of emergency. Purchase the deluxe organizer ($40) or paperback bound workbook ($25) from Planet Media Group HealthHistory.com at 4245 Watermill Ave. Orlando, FL 32817; 877-907-9494; www. HealthHistory.com.

• • • • • • • • • • • • • • • • • • • • • • • •

**Wear a MedicAlert® bracelet** if you have a serious medical condition. Especially important for someone who would have difficulty remembering a serious medical condition, the MedicAlert® bracelet alerts medical professionals to allergies and medical conditions (diabetes, epilepsy, heart disease, etc.) that require special attention. Ask your pharmacist about ordering or contact the MedicAlert® Foundation International, 2323 Colorado Avenue, Turlock, CA 95382; 888-633-4298; www.medicalert.org.

• • • • • • • • • • • • • • • • • • • • • • • •

**The MEDLINEplus health information site,** run by the National Institutes of Health (NIH), explains medical terms in everyday language. If you don't understand information in your medical records or cannot remember what a prescription is for, go to www.nlm.nih.gov/medlineplus.

• • • • • • • • • • • • • • • • • • • • • • • • •

**Learn about treatment options** with the help of the NIH. Considered to represent state-of-the-art treatment guidelines in medical practice, the NIH can help you keep details of your medical condition straight, get a second opinion, compare recommendations and be confident that you have the information you need to make educated decisions.

• • • • • • • • • • • • • • • • • • • • • • • • •

**Focus on the positive** by keeping a progress calendar. Mark the calendar with stickers and encouraging comments each day. When a bad day comes around, you can remind yourself or the person you care for of the good things.

## Learning about medications

**Medication side effects** can mimic memory loss. If you are suddenly having difficulty remembering things and have changed medication or medical therapies recently, discuss the situation with your doctor. Sometimes a minor change in medication can make a big difference in your life.

• • • • • • • • • • • • • • • • • • • • • • • • •

**Compare notes with your pharmacist.** Ask your pharmacist for written instructions and a list of side effects for any medication your doctor prescribes. If you are still confused or the doctor's and the pharmacist's instructions differ, consult the *USP DI Advice for the Patient: Drug Information in Lay Language, Volume II,* at your local library. Or simply Google the specific medication. If you still have questions, contact your doctor for an explanation.

• • • • • • • • • • • • • • • • • • • • • • • • •

**Know medical abbreviations.** Do all those Latin abbreviations confuse you? To help you remember what b.i.d., t.i.d and q.i.d. stand for, think of them this way: "Bi" has two letters, "tri" has three and "quad" has four. So take a medication marked "b.i.d" twice a day, "t.i.d." three times a day and "q.i.d." four times a day.

• • • • • • • • • • • • • • • • • • • • • • • • •

**Make sure medications are fresh.** Medications can become ineffective or even dangerous when they get old. When the seasons change, take a few moments to check the expiration dates of your medications, discard outdated ones and make a list of those that need to be refilled.

• • • • • • • • • • • • • • • • • • • • • • • • •

**Write a note** regarding why the medication was prescribed. When you get home with a new medication, write in your notebook or on the label what the drug is for to remind you to use it only for the prescribed condition.

• • • • • • • • • • • • • • • • • • • • • • • • •

**Sign up for automatic drug refills** through a mail-order pharmacy. Afraid you'll forget to pick up your prescriptions? Ask if the pharmacy offers automatic reminder calls or sends email messages to let you know your prescriptions are ready.

• • • • • • • • • • • • • • • • • • • • •

**Place a standing order with the pharmacy** for easy-open containers and you won't have to remind the pharmacist again. (Remember, these containers are not childproof and may pose a health risk to children and confused adults.) You may also want to request large-print labels, detailed instructions or whatever else would be helpful.

• • • • • • • • • • • • • • • • • • • • •

**Keep extra doses of medication** in your wallet or purse in case you forget to take your medication before you leave for the day or you need extra medication before you get home.

• • • • • • • • • • • • • • • • • • • • •

**Take copies of your prescriptions** with you when you travel. If you drop, lose or misplace your medication, you can have it refilled easily. Make sure your physician knows you're going away and writes the prescription to cover enough medication for your trip.

• • • • • • • • • • • • • • • • • • • • •

**Have your prescriptions filled** by a national pharmacy. If you forget your meds when traveling, your stay is extended or you have miscalculated what you need, you'll have easy access to refills.

• • • • • • • • • • • • • • • • • • • • •

# Organizing medications

**Prepackage your daily medications.** Keep track of daily medications by lining up all your pill bottles on the counter, labeling self-sealing plastic sandwich bags with the days of the week and then packaging your daily medications in the appropriate bag.

**Separate your daily medication dose** in the bottle. To help you remember if you have taken your medication, try this: From each bottle, remove the cotton and take out the number of pills you'll need for the day. Then replace the cotton and set the selected pills on top of the cotton. Replace the cap. Pills will stay in their original container, and you can tell at a glance whether you have taken your daily dose.

**Use a seven-day pill organizer** to keep track of medications. If you take several prescriptions, some every day, some every other day, some in the morning and some at bedtime, the seven-day pill organizer may be helpful in reminding you when to take each medication. The organizer has seven daily cases, each with four separate compartments for morning, noon, evening and bedtime medications. All seven cases fit into a tray, and each daily container snaps out to carry in your pocket. e-pill® Medication Reminders, e-pill, LLC, 70 Walnut Street, Wellesley, MA 02481; 800-549-0095; www.epill.com.

**The Talking Rx™ reminds you** of prescription use and dosage. This device allows you, your pharmacist or a family member to easily record a spoken message with instructions on how and when to take the medication. To hear the dosage instructions, you simply press the red button on the lid. Talking Rx™ is also helpful for those who have difficulty reading the tiny print on medicine bottles or understanding English print. $20. Easy Street Co., 384 Wickham Road, North Kingstown, RI 02852; 800-959-3279; www.easystreetco.com.

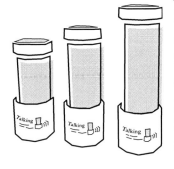

**Have a pharmacist or visiting nurse** divide up your pills if you have difficulty remembering your daily medication dose.

# Remembering to take medication

**Create a daily medication schedule** with boxes for noting each medication and when to take it. Keep the schedule handy and check off each dosage as you take it. For extra assurance, tape the schedule for each medication to the bottle. A printed schedule is especially important when you are unable to medicate yourself or unable to tell someone else when your next dose is due. Ask your doctor if you can simplify your schedule so you're taking all or most of your medications once or twice a day.

**Track your medication schedule** on a bulletin board to help you see what meds to take at what time. Write the times of day on separate pieces of paper or cardstock and tack in chronological order across the top of the board. Write and tack the days of the week down the left side of the board. Fill clear, self-sealing plastic bags with the correct dose of medication for each specific time of day and tack the bags to the bulletin board under the appropriate day and time, adding instructions such as "drink plenty of water" or "take with food." You can tell at a glance when to take your medication and if you have forgotten a dose. Of course, the bulletin board should be kept out of the reach of children and those who aren't mentally alert. Medications that should not be exposed directly to light can be wrapped in a small amount of aluminum foil before placing them in the bag.

• • • • • • • • • • • • • • • • • • • • • • • • •

**Put your morning medication** in your slipper. To remember to take a medication first thing in the morning, put the pill bottle in your slipper. Before you can put on your slippers, you'll have to remove the pill bottle. Take the medication with a glass of water you keep on your nightstand.

• • • • • • • • • • • • • • • • • • • • • • • • •

**Keep morning meds and a glass of water** at your bedside to remember to take your medications first thing in the morning. If you're taking pain medication, you may want to wake up earlier than necessary to take the medication and then go back to sleep until it begins working.

• • • • • • • • • • • • • • • • • • • • • • • • •

**To remember to take a medication** first thing in the morning, place the pill bottle somewhere you will see it. If you start the day with a cup of coffee, put your medication inside your favorite coffee cup or on top of the coffee sweetener. Don't drink coffee? Put your pills or pill bottle in your favorite cereal bowl or near the pet food where a hungry pet can remind you to take your morning medication.

• • • • • • • • • • • • • • • • • • • • • • • • • •

**Keep medications handy** in a decorative container. Place the container on the kitchen table or near a favorite chair or couch where it will remind you to take your meds, while eliminating the unsightliness of all those bottles. Of course, keep all medications out of their reach if there are children in the house.

• • • • • • • • • • • • • • • • • • • • • • • • • •

**Use the alphabet to remember** whether you should take your medications in the morning or evening. Assign each medication an "a" if it is taken in the morning (a.m.) or a "p" if it is taken at night (p.m.). ("A" comes before "p" in the alphabet.)

• • • • • • • • • • • • • • • • • • • • • • • • • •

**Consider time-release medications.** Many medications come in long-acting or time-release versions. With fewer doses, you have less to remember and fewer pills to take. Ask your doctor if a long-acting or time-release version is appropriate for you.

• • • • • • • • • • • • • • • • • • • • • • • • • •

# Injections

### Use hand tracing to record injection sites.
If you are diabetic and have difficulty remembering which fingers have been used for blood sugar monitoring, trace an outline of a pair of hands on a piece of paper and mark the site of the last blood sample. This will help you remember to change sites.

• • • • • • • • • • • • • • • • • • • • • • • • • • • •

### Use a bracelet to remember to alternate injection locations.
If you need to alternate injection sites and have trouble remembering which side you did last, wear a bracelet on the arm where the injection went. When you give the next injection, move the bracelet to the other arm. If you don't like to wear bracelets, change a ring from one hand to the other or use a sticky tab on the medication that indicates right or left. If the medication is refrigerated, you may want to use a refrigerator magnet to help you remember which side, arm or leg to use.

• • • • • • • • • • • • • • • • • • • • • • • • • • • •

### Mark syringes with the correct dose of injectable medication.
If it is difficult to remember the proper dosage for insulin or other injectable medications, use a marking pen or dab of colored nail polish to mark the correct level on each syringe.

• • • • • • • • • • • • • • • • • • • • • • • • • • • •

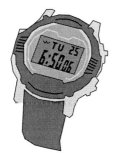

### The MeDose™ medication reminder watch

reminds you to take meds. The watch looks like a normal sports watch but uses vibration or sound to remind you to take medicine. It has six alarms, an auto-reset timer, and day-date and stopwatch functions. 800-549-0095; www.epill.com.

• • • • • • • • • • • • • • • • • • • • • • • •

### The MedGlider™ System pillbox with alarm

reminds you when to take medications. This electronic timer has three types of alarms (beeping, voice, visual), which remind you up to three times at one-minute intervals. The large, easy-to-read LCD screen displays the current time and the number of daily doses (up to four). It has large buttons and separate hour and minute buttons for easy programming. The MedGlider™ timer can be attached to a four-compartment pillbox and is small enough to fit in a coat pocket. e-pill® Medication Reminders, e-pill, LLC, 70 Walnut Street, Wellesley, MA 02481; 800-549-0095; www.epill.com.

• • • • • • • • • • • • • • • • • • • • • • • •

### Use a digital sports watch timer to remind

you to take meds every two, four or six hours. For example, set the timer to beep after four hours. Once it beeps, it automatically starts counting down to the next four-hour interval. These watches come in men and women's styles with metal or nylon bands.

• • • • • • • • • • • • • • • • • • • • • • • •

# Scheduling appointments

**Schedule annual appointments** (physicals, eye exams, mammograms, etc.) around annual events such as birthdays or anniversaries to help you remember your appointment. Choose a time of year that is less busy for both you and your doctor.

• • • • • • • • • • • • • • • • • • • • • • • • •

**Mark your calendar** to schedule long-range appointments. If you are seeing a specialist and it takes weeks or months to schedule an appointment, enter the reminder information on your calendar two to three months before you need to see the doctor.

• • • • • • • • • • • • • • • • • • • • • • • • •

**Have your doctor's receptionist** write the date and time of your next appointment on a business or appointment card. If you must change the appointment, you'll have the phone number handy. This tip works well any place you make return or follow-up appointments.

• • • • • • • • • • • • • • • • • • • • • • • • •

**Temporarily record an appointment** on the palm of your hand. Don't have a business card or calendar with you to record the date? Write the date in the palm of your hand to remember until you get home and can write it on your calendar.

• • • • • • • • • • • • • • • • • • • • • • • • •

**Ask your doctor's office to remind you** of an appointment by sending you a reminder letter or calling you a day or two before your appointment. You could also ask for a reminder note to make a six-month dental checkup, an annual mammogram or a two-year colonoscopy.

# Communicating with professionals

### Be honest about your medical history.
Your doctors can act only on what you tell them. If you are not completely honest with medical professionals, they will not have all the information they need to treat you properly. Be sure to inform them of all the symptoms you're having, no matter how minor or silly they might seem. Also remind them of all current prescription medications, even if they prescribed them, as well as over-the-counter drugs and supplements. Doctors who don't have all the facts will find it difficult to diagnose and treat you properly.

• • • • • • • • • • • • • • • • • • • • • • • • • •

**Compile a list of questions** before doctors' appointments. Put each of your doctors' names on an envelope and store the envelopes in an easily accessible spot. When you think of a question you want to ask a specific doctor, write it down and place it in the appropriate envelope. The day before your next appointment, prepare a written list of questions. Be sure to prioritize your list so you ask the most important questions first.

• • • • • • • • • • • • • • • • • • • • • • • • • •

**Ask for videotaped instructions** for special procedures to perform at home. If you have difficulty remembering how to do a special procedure or technique ordered by the doctor, ask the nursing staff if they will make a videotape to show you what needs to be done. They might also explain the reason for the procedures and possible complications. If a videotape is not feasible, you might create a photo book with simple explanations illustrated by pictures of equipment, procedures and so forth.

• • • • • • • • • • • • • • • • • • • • • • • • • • • •

**Take along plain self-adhesive labels** when you go to the doctor's office. If your doctor prescribes medication, write down what the doctor tells you and stick it on the bottle when you get the prescription filled.

# Finding support

**Contact national health organizations** for helpful information. If a family member's memory is affected by an illness such as MS, Parkinson's or Alzheimer's, you may find helpful information by contacting the national organization for the specific illness. Consult your librarian for a list of organizations and their contact information.

• • • • • • • • • • • • • • • • • • • • • • • • • • • •

**A national network** of independent living centers can put you in touch with vital support and services. Every community in the United States is part of a national network of more than 500 independent living centers (ILC). These community-based, nonprofit centers serve people of all ages and disabilities and their families. They can help you find out about disability services in your community, connect you with others to advocate for changes in the law or rules, help you hire and manage personal care attendants and put you in contact with people who have faced challenges similar to your own. For a national directory of independent living centers, contact the National Council on Independent Living, 1916 Wilson Boulevard, Suite 209, Arlington, VA 22201; 703-525-3406; TTY: 703-525-4153; fax: 703-525-3409; www.ncil.org.

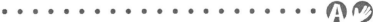

## Seek out assistance from social workers.

If you or a loved one has been diagnosed with a chronic medical condition or disability, consult a social worker, who can help you connect with supportive services in your community. Social workers often work in rehab centers and hospitals, where they do discharge planning. You will also find them in community service agencies such as Catholic, Lutheran or Jewish social services.

**Find a list of area resources** at ElderCarelink. If your loved one's memory causes you concerns, perhaps you're considering hiring caregivers. ElderCarelink can provide a list of knowledgeable and qualified providers that can meet the needs of your family. www.eldercarelink.com. 🅐 🖐

# Helping others

**Keep a daily diary** and communication notebook. When several family members are caring for a loved one, at home or in a facility, keep a binder or notebook to make notes, communicate messages and record information regarding symptoms, medications, dates of illnesses or procedures. While keeping everyone informed of changes on a daily basis, your notebook will help you remember little details that may be important later.

• • • • • • • • • • • • • • • • • • • • • • • • 🅐 🖐

**Post special instructions** in a prominent place. If you have specific instructions for caring for a wound, changing a catheter or moving a loved one in bed, type or write the instructions in large block letters on 8" x 10" cardstock. Place the instruction card in an easel-type picture frame and post in a prominent place where everyone can see and follow the instructions.

• • • • • • • • • • • • • • • • • • • • • • • • 🅐 🖐

**Create step-by-step instructions.** A change in routine can be very distressing for someone with severe memory loss. If you perform certain caregiving tasks infrequently, write down step-by-step instructions, illustrated with pictures, and post above your loved one's bed. You and anyone who shares the caregiving tasks can easily follow the instructions, assuring greater comfort and continuity of care for the confused person.

• • • • • • • • • • • • • • • • • • • • • • •

**To remember the warning signs** of a stroke, you might find this mnemonic helpful: **W**e k**N**ow the **H**ints to a **P**ossible **S**troke; we can **S**ee the **D**ifference. This will help you remember to be on the lookout for Weakness, Numbness, Headache, Personality changes, Speech changes, Sight changes and Dizziness.

• • • • • • • • • • • • • • • • • • • • • • •

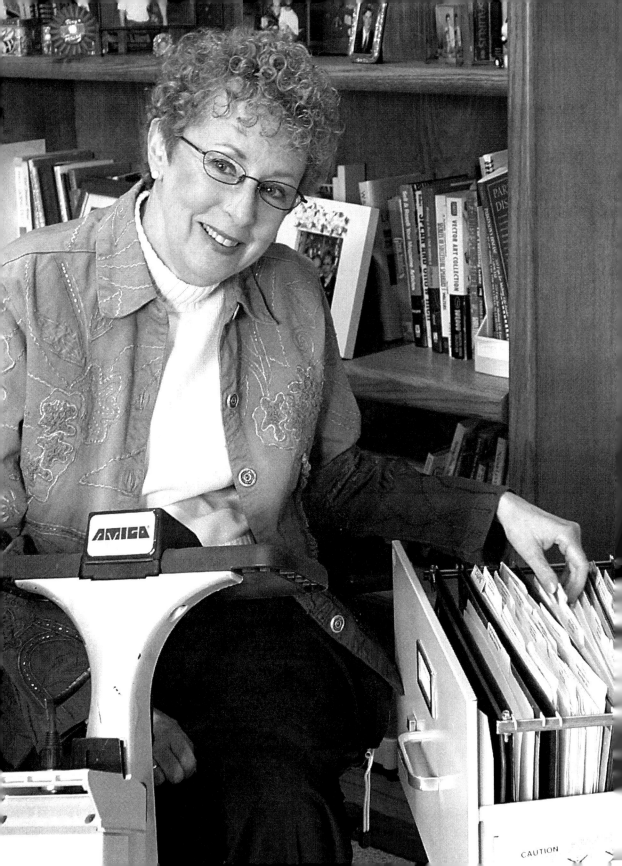

# 7

# taking care
# of business

Remembering what needs to be done, finding stores and services, running errands and paying bills in an organized way are things we deal with, if not every day, at least every month. I have found that using the ideas in this chapter has changed not only my life but the lives of my husband and children as well. Now that my children are adults, I'm proud to say they rarely forget to pay a bill, miss a birthday or get lost when looking for a new address. I like to think these tips have helped them as I hope they'll help you.

# ASSESSING YOUR NEEDS

**To get organized, it would be helpful to:**

- ○ Limit errands to one or two at a time
- ○ Plan the route for errand trips
- ○ Create a book of personal travel directions
- ○ Keep track of addresses in a small photo album
- ○ Keep an extra phone book in the trunk

**To run errands more easily, it would be helpful to:**

- ○ Use a fictitious phone number to remember my PIN
- ○ Use a checkbook with duplicate checks
- ○ Mark the last three checks to remember to refill the checkbook
- ○ Look for ATMs with no surcharge
- ○ Arrange for automatic withdrawal to pay bills
- ○ Use contact numbers on bills to confirm payment
- ○ Write the check number on each receipt
- ○ Keep track of library due dates
- ○ Place library books by the door when due
- ○ Write appointments on business cards
- ○ Use a grocery store map
- ○ Shop on Tuesdays
- ○ Ask for building directions
- ○ Tie a ribbon on the car antenna
- ○ Staple business cards to product information
- ○ Take a picture to jog my memory
- ○ Take swatches and paint samples when shopping
- ○ Create a gift list with sizes, addresses, etc.
- ○ Use picture communication cards

**To make driving easier, it would be helpful to:**

○ Establish a routine for leaving the car
○ Keep important papers in the glove compartment
○ Change one small thing to jog the memory
○ Use sticky notes to remember errands
○ Clip notes to the visor
○ Keep a calendar handy for alternate parking dates
○ Write a note with parking location information
○ Locate the car with the panic button
○ Use a parking timer to mind the meter
○ Purchase a portable jump starter

# Organizing yourself

**Limit errands to one or two at a time** if remembering a sequence of four or five errands is too frustrating or tiring. After one or two errands, go home and get organized for the next set of errands. Go out again when you feel rested.

• • • • • • • • • • • • • • • • • • • • • • • • • • •

**Think over the route for the stops** on your errand trips and write it down if you are prone to forgetting the sequence. Before you leave home, consider: Is this a good time of day to be going to the library or post office? Will the drive-up windows at the bank be open? Will there be lines? Rearrange the sequence of stops to make it most convenient for you.

• • • • • • • • • • • • • • • • • • • • • • • • • • •

**Create a book** of personal travel directions. If you find it difficult to remember how to get to specific places around town, create a personal travel directions booklet. Purchase a small (4" x 6") photo album, found at drug, discount and photo developing stores. Fill the pages with directions to the library, dry cleaners and other places you may have difficulty finding. This works well for long distance travel as well. Create a page for each family member or destination. Include a list of frequently used telephone numbers and directions or maps to grocery stores, shopping malls, parks, schools and houses of worship.

• • • • • • • • • • • • • • • • • • • • • • • • • • •

**Keep track of addresses, maps and more** in a small photo album. A small plastic photo album is a great way to keep track of addresses, phone numbers, directions and maps. Write all pertinent information on index cards and tuck the cards into the photo pockets. Your album stores neatly in the glove compartment, ready at a moment's notice if you lose your way or need to remember a name or phone number.

• • • • • • • • • • • • • • • • • • • • • • • • • •

**An extra phone book stored in the trunk** of your car can be a ready reference for locating addresses and telephone numbers.

## Running errands

**Use a fictitious phone number** to remember your Personal Identification Number (PIN) for your bank card or credit card. Make the last four numbers of the phone number your PIN and write the number in a notebook that you carry in your purse or organizer.

• • • • • • • • • • • • • • • • • • • • • • • • • •

**Avoid omissions in your checkbook register** by using duplicate checks. If you forget to write in the amount, the duplicate is in your checkbook for handy reference. Sign up for overdraft protection for those times when you record a deposit twice or goof up the math.

• • • • • • • • • • • • • • • • • • • • • • • • • •

**Mark your last three checks** to remember to refill your checkbook. On the last check put a small "0" in the corner, on the one before that a "1" and on the one before that a "2." You'll know when you get to the last three checks.

• • • • • • • • • • • • • • • • • • • • • • • • •

**Look for ATMs with no surcharge.** If you forget to stop at the bank and run out of money frequently, ATM charges can really add up. Look for ATMs with a "No Surcharge Here" sign—most often found at local credit unions and grocery stores.

• • • • • • • • • • • • • • • • • • • • • • • • •

**Consider an automatic withdrawal plan** to pay bills. If you dislike writing checks to pay the bills, consider an automatic withdrawal payment plan. Each month your bill is paid automatically through your checking account, so you never miss a payment or pay a late fee. If you prefer to stay in charge of your bill paying, sign up for an Internet bill paying account at your bank and set your computer to remind you to pay bills on certain days. Either way, there's the added benefit of no cost for checks, envelopes or stamps, not to mention the time you save.

• • • • • • • • • • • • • • • • • • • • • • • • •

**Use contact numbers on bills** to confirm payment. Can't remember if you've paid a bill? Often the telephone number of the payment department is listed on the front or back of the bill. You might also sign up for an Internet account and check online anytime, day or night.

• • • • • • • • • • • • • • • • • • • • • • • • •

## Write your check number on your receipt.

If you carry a single check rather than your checkbook, make sure you remember to record it in the check register by writing the check number on the purchase receipt. If you get in the habit of doing this every time you write a check, with or without your checkbook, you'll always have a record of your transaction.

• • • • • • • • • • • • • • • • • • • • • • • • • •

## Keep track of library book return dates.

Many libraries now give you a small, easy-to-lose receipt instead of stamping your book with the return date. To help you remember the return date, write it on the old return slip inside the book. If your book does not have one, write the date on a sticky note and place it inside the front cover. If your receipt gets lost, you'll know when to return the books. Missed a library due date? Some libraries don't fine seniors and some waive the overdue fines for all their patrons. Inquire.

• • • • • • • • • • • • • • • • • • • • • • • • • •

## Place library books by your door when due.

If you're afraid you'll forget to return library books that are due, put them on the floor in front of the door. You won't leave home without seeing the books and remembering to take them. Use the same strategy to remember to take other items when you leave.

• • • • • • • • • • • • • • • • • • • • • • • • • •

**When making a hair appointment,** have the receptionist write the appointment date and time on an appointment reminder card or business card with the business name and phone number on it. If you must change the appointment, you'll have the number handy. This works well for medical offices or any other place you make return or follow-up appointments.

• • • • • • • • • • • • • • • • • • • • • • • •

**Obtain a map of your grocery store** and write your grocery list by aisle. An organized list will help you avoid backtracking, buying on impulse or forgetting items.

• • • • • • • • • • • • • • • • • • • • • • • •

**Shop on Tuesdays.** If you find shopping to be distracting and chaotic, try going on Tuesdays. According to a survey by a national grocery association, Tuesday is the least busy day of the week.

• • • • • • • • • • • • • • • • • • • • • • • •

**Ask for directions immediately.** When entering large facilities like department stores, libraries and shopping centers, ask for directions immediately. This keeps you from getting lost and saves time and energy. Often store maps or layouts are available for visitors.

• • • • • • • • • • • • • • • • • • • • • • • •

**Tie a bright ribbon** on your car radio antenna to help locate your car quickly in large grocery or mall parking lots. Another way to help locate your car in a parking lot is to put a colorful hat or stuffed animal on the back shelf of your car. You'll be able to distinguish your car from the others more easily.

• • • • • • • • • • • • • • • • • • • • • • • •

**Staple business cards to product information.** When shopping for furniture, appliances or a vehicle, you may visit several stores and talk with several salespeople. For a handy reference when you're ready to make a purchase, staple the salesperson's business card to any product information. Note on the back of the card a description of the store or the salesperson and any other information that will help you jog your memory to differentiate vendors. This technique also comes in handy when dealing with medical information from doctors and with operating manuals, invoices, warranty information or any other specific information you want to connect to a person.

• • • • • • • • • • • • • • • • • • • • • • • •

**Take your digital camera with you** when you shop for furniture, a vehicle, a house—any big-ticket item you would shop around for. When you get home, the pictures, along with your notes, will help you remember which was which.

• • • • • • • • • • • • • • • • • • • • • • • •

**Keep a swatch of paint** with your decorating materials so you have it for color comparison when shopping. You can use a paint chip from the store or create your own larger one by painting on white cardboard. This has the added advantage of allowing you to have a larger sample of the paint to compare with whatever it is you're matching—wall color, carpet, upholstery, etc.

• • • • • • • • • • • • • • • • • • • • • • • • • • •

**Record personal information on a gift list.**
To remember the sizes and measurements of people on your gift-buying list, keep them on a piece of paper in your purse or wallet. Having out-of-state addresses with you could also save time and energy. Let the store wrap and mail gifts directly to the recipients.

• • • • • • • • • • • • • • • • • • • • • • • • • • •

**Shopping cards.** For those who have trouble remembering the right word when shopping, picture cards may help them communicate their needs. These brightly colored, laminated cards have pictures that depict common words and items. Shoppers can simply select the appropriate card for the word they want to say when their memory fails. Other sets of picture communication cards are available for home and activities. About $49/set. Attainment Company, Inc., PO Box 930160, Verona, WI 53593-0160; 800-327-4269; fax: 800-942-3865; www.AttainmentCompany.com.

• • • • • • • • • • • • • • • • • • • • • • •

# Driving

**Establish a pattern for safety** and peace of mind. Have you ever gotten out of your car, walked away and then had to go back to check that you locked it? If so, create a routine that you go through every time you leave your vehicle: Shut off the lights, secure the parking brake, lock the car doors and then double check the lights, brake and locks before you walk away. You might even tell yourself the car is secure. Following a specific routine and telling yourself you're doing each step will imprint the action on your mind.

• • • • • • • • • • • • • • • • • • • • • • • •

**Keep a large envelope** in the glove compartment of your car and put receipts for new tires, oil changes, tune-ups and batteries inside. Write the dates of your last tune-up, oil change or tire rotation on the outside of the envelope so you'll know at a glance when your car is due for these services again. At the end of the year, transfer the last service dates to a new envelope and file the envelope in your automotive file by year. If you don't need records for income tax or other purposes, separate out the major repairs and warranties and discard the rest.

• • • • • • • • • • • • • • • • • • • • • • • •

**Jog your memory by putting your purse** or briefcase in the back seat. If you think of something you want to remember while driving the car, reach over (safely, of course!) and put your purse or briefcase in the back seat. When you don't find it in its usual place when you park, it triggers your memory. Other things you might do: Move your wedding ring, bracelet or watch to the opposite hand or push the sun visor down. The idea is to change the familiar to something unfamiliar to remind yourself that you want to remember something.

· · · · · · · · · · · · · · · · · · · · · · · · · · · · · ·

**To remember all your errands** while you're out, write the list on a sticky note, put it on the dashboard and check off the errands as you do them. If this is still too far out of sight and thus out of mind, put your list near the speedometer so when you check your speed you're reminded of what you have to do.

· · · · · · · · · · · · · · · · · · · · · · · · · · · · · ·

**Clip notes to the sun visor of your vehicle.** If you have a tendency to misplace things in the car (to-do list, directions, parking garage tickets, dry cleaning claim tickets and other loose pieces of paper), clip the items to the sun visor with clothespins or binder clips. If you make this a habit, you'll remember what you have to do, your car will be more organized and you'll save time searching for items.

· · · · · · · · · · · · · · · · · · · · · · · · · · · · · ·

**Track alternate side parking** with a small calendar in your car to help you remember whether it's an even or odd day. Wallet cards can be attached to the visor with hook and loop fastener tape.

• • • • • • • • • • • • • • • • • • • • • • • • • • •

**Keep notepaper and a pen in your pocket** to jot down where you parked your car. For example, write down the number of parking spaces to the main aisle. If you park in an unpaved area with few landmarks, find a tree, sign or other distinctive marker and add that to your parking notes.

• • • • • • • • • • • • • • • • • • • • • • • • • • •

**Activate your car's panic button** to help you locate your car in a large parking lot.

• • • • • • • • • • • • • • • • • • • • • • • • • • •

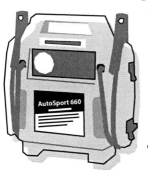

**A parking timer minds the meter,** keeps the deadline and remembers where you parked! The device can also be used to remember appointments. About $25. Sharper Image; 800-344-5555; www.sharperimage.com.

• • • • • • • • • • • • • • • • • • • • • • • • • • •

**Purchase a portable jump starter.** If you tend to run down your car battery by forgetting to turn off the lights, a portable jump starter can have you quickly on your way without calling an auto club. Driving Comfort.com, PO Box 9036, Charlottesville, VA 22906; 800-675-5411; www.drivingcomfort.com.

• • • • • • • • • • • • • • • • • • • • • • • • • • •

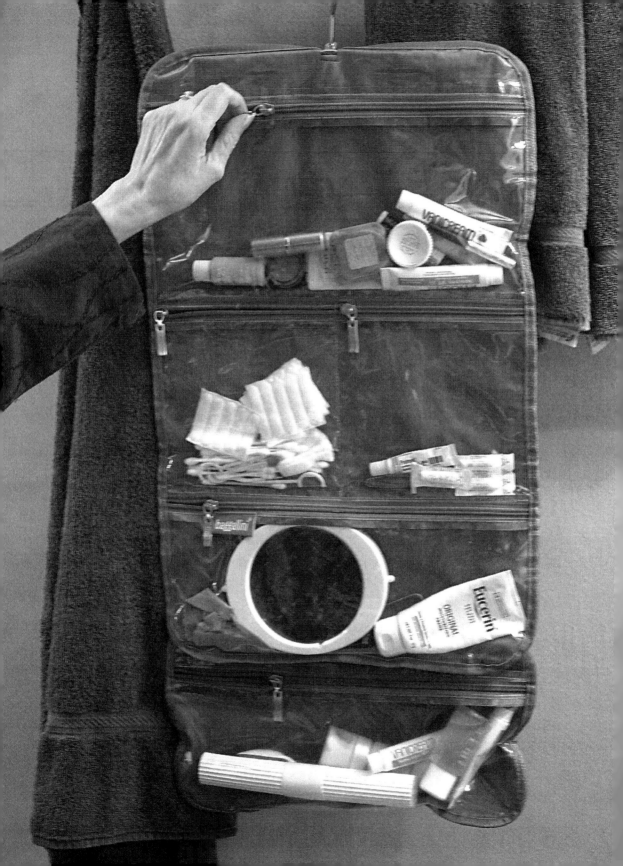

# 8

# travel

I love to travel but getting ready for a trip, however long or short, creates stress. There are so many details to remember. I've learned lots of tips that have helped me leave the comforts of my home without worrying that I have forgotten something. By creating a travel folder with copies of all the lists and reminders I use whenever we go away, I rarely forget to cancel the newspaper, turn down the hot water heater or grind up the food in the garbage disposal before we leave.

# ASSESSING YOUR NEEDS

**To prepare for a trip, it would be helpful to:**

◯ Create a "What to take with me" list

◯ Create a "What to do before I leave" list

◯ Compile a list of the important information to take on the trip

◯ Make a list of emergency contact and medical information

◯ Document travel plans with names and numbers

◯ Set up automatic bill paying

◯ Arrange for a wake-up call

**When packing, it would be helpful to:**

◯ Laminate an all-purpose packing list

◯ Select a place to gather travel items prior to packing

◯ Keep a packing checklist

**To travel safely, it would be helpful to:**

◯ Eat right, exercise and get enough sleep

◯ Make photocopies of important documents

◯ Photocopy both sides of credit cards

◯ Organize travel information in a file

◯ Attach earrings to watchband

**To travel by plane or train, it would be helpful to:**

○ Write a detailed itinerary and information list
○ Attach travel information to a carry-on
○ Be aware of what my traveling companion is wearing
○ Inquire about a special pass to accompany a passenger to the gate

**To make driving easier, it would be helpful to:**

○ Understand the Interstate highway numbering system
○ Keep toll money in a container
○ Obtain an electronic tollway pass

**To remember trips, it would be helpful to:**

○ Take along pre-addressed address labels
○ Write thank-you notes while traveling
○ Write down memories as I go

# Remembering everything

**Create a packing list.** Include the obvious: Clothing, accessories, toiletries and so forth. Also include the not-so-obvious: Trip information (maps, itinerary, passports), address book, stamps for postcards, laundry bag (for dirty clothes), extra canvas bag (for purchases) and fun stuff (games, reading material, sporting equipment). Each family member may want to create an individual list.

• • • • • • • • • • • • • • • • • • • • • • • • • •

**Write a list of things that can be done** a few days before you leave: Get substitute drivers for carpools, cancel lessons, find someone to mow the lawn (or shovel snow), arrange for newspaper and mail pick-up and leave a key and itinerary (with phone numbers) with neighbors. For car trips, add: Check air in tires (including spare), purchase snack foods for cooler and put selected tools in trunk in case of an emergency.

• • • • • • • • • • • • • • • • • • • • • • • • • •

**List things to do right before you leave:** Set the heat or air conditioning to conserve energy; turn down the hot water heater; unplug all appliances; empty the refrigerator of perishables; grind up anything left in the garbage disposal; take out the garbage; set automatic timers on lights, radio or TV; adjust the shades or blinds to look like someone is home; park a car in the driveway (or arrange for a neighbor to park there); and check to see that all the doors are locked.

• • • • • • • • • • • • • • • • • • • • • • • • • • •

**Compile a list of the important information** you need to take on your trip: Numbers on important documents (driver's license, passport, etc.); phone numbers for family, airlines, credit card companies and the American Embassy; and your travel itinerary. Print the information in a small font size, laminate it and clip it in your wallet. For added security, leave a copy in a file at home and with the person watching your home.

• • • • • • • • • • • • • • • • • • • • • • • • • • •

**Make a list of emergency contact** and medical information. Include the names of the medications you're taking, the dosage, time of day you take the drug, what it is for and how long you have been taking it. (Don't forget to include any allergies you have to medications, preservatives, etc.) Also list the names and telephone numbers of family members or close friends who should be contacted in case of emergency as well as your doctors, therapists, counselors, hospitals and clinics. Print the information in a small font size, laminate it and keep with your passport or driver's license in your wallet or purse. If you are traveling to a foreign country, check with a local university language department about having this information translated into the language of your destination country. Give a copy to your spouse or traveling companion in case yours is lost or stolen.

• • • • • • • • • • • • • • • • • • • • • • • • • • • •

**Make written notes of travel plans.** Always take notes when making travel plans over the phone. Should something go wrong or there is any question later, you'll have a record, in writing, of whom you spoke with and what was said (promises, rates, etc.).

• • • • • • • • • • • • • • • • • • • • • • • • • • • •

**Pay bills automatically.** If you'll be gone from home for an extended time, one way to remember to pay your bills is to arrange to have them paid automatically. A month or two before the trip, arrange to put your utility bills (gas and electric, telephone, cell phone, cable, etc.) on autopay. Once your account is set up, the monthly payment is automatically taken directly out of your checking account. Of course, you can use this service all year round if you desire.

• • • • • • • • • • • • • • • • • • • • • • • • • • • • •

**Arrange for a wake-up call.** When traveling, ask the hotel to give you a wake-up call so you don't miss an appointment or commitment. If you travel a great deal and are concerned you might forget to set your alarm or request a hotel wake-up call, arrange for a service provided by www.wakeupland.com. You schedule the time you want to receive wake-up calls and the phone number to call.

# Packing

**Laminate an all-purpose list** of things you pack in your suitcase. Use an erasable marker to check things off as you pack. When you finish packing, wipe off the list and store it in your travel file. If you need to add additional items unique to a trip, put a sticky note on the laminated list.

• • • • • • • • • • • • • • • • • • • • • • • • • • • • •

**Select a place to gather travel items** prior to packing. As you remember things that aren't on your general packing list (gifts, cards, camera bag, extra medication, etc.), put them in this place so you'll remember them when you pack your bags.

• • • • • • • • • • • • • • • • • • • • • • • • • • • •

**Keep a packing checklist** permanently inside your suitcase. Add to the list as your travel destinations change.

## Traveling safely

**Take care of yourself.** Keep your memory in good working order while you are traveling by eating well, getting plenty of exercise and sleeping on a regular schedule.

• • • • • • • • • • • • • • • • • • • • • • • • • • • •

**Travel with photocopies** of important documents. If you are traveling overseas, take a photocopy of your passport and two extra passport photos with you and keep them separate from your original passport. If your passport is lost or stolen, you'll have what you need to replace it. It may also be a good idea to copy your airline ticket, traveler's checks and driver's license. Keep one set for yourself, away from the originals; leave one set with a friend or family member; and keep another in the hotel safe at your destination.

• • • • • • • • • • • • • • • • • • • • • • • • • • • •

**Make photocopies of both sides** of your credit cards. Keep one in a file at home, give your spouse a copy and leave one in a safe place away from your card when you travel. If you lose a card, it'll be easy to report. (The phone number to report your loss is on the back of each card.)

• • • • • • • • • • • • • • • • • • • • • • • • • •

**Keep travel information organized in a file.** For long trips, use a file organizer with divider tabs to keep all your travel information together in one place. Dividers might include hotel (address, phone number, confirmation information), car rental, travel documents (copies of passport, tickets), destination information (maps, travel brochures, articles) and phone cards. Keep the file organizer in your carry-on bag and everything will be accessible when you need it.

• • • • • • • • • • • • • • • • • • • • • • • • • •

**Attach your earrings to your watchband.** When traveling, attach your earrings to your watchband to make sure you don't accidentally leave them on the nightstand when you leave your hotel room. Fasten posts, wires or hoops through the holes in the band or snap clip-ons to the band.

• • • • • • • • • • • • • • • • • • • • • • • • • •

# Planes, trains, buses, ships

**Ease travel confusion** with a detailed itinerary and information list. If a person is easily confused, create a detailed travel itinerary and information list to consult when traveling. Include the date, flight (train, bus) information, transfer or connection information, home address, family and emergency contact information and who will be meeting the person at the end of the ride. Preparing this information will prevent unnecessary anxiety on the part of the traveler and ease the minds of family members on either end.

**Attach travel information to your carry-on.** When you travel, attach a tag to your carry-on bag that indicates your flight numbers, departure times and seat assignments. Then put your tickets safely away in your bag until you need them to get through security.

**Take note of what your traveling companion** is wearing. Airports, railway and bus stations, ships, trains and even large aircraft are usually busy and confusing places where it's easy to lose touch with a traveling companion. Always take note of what your companion is wearing. It can also be useful to carry a recent photograph of them.

**Inquire about a special pass** to accompany a passenger to the gate. For someone who may become easily confused or forgetful, making it difficult to locate the right gate without assistance, explain to the ticket agent at the time of check-in that you would like to accompany the passenger to the proper gate and why. It's common practice for ticket agents to issue a special pass that will allow someone to guide a ticketed passenger through security and get them safely on the plane. You'll need a picture ID and must go through security just like passengers with tickets.

## Automobiles

**The Interstate highway numbering system** can keep you from going the wrong direction. Remember that odd numbered highways travel north and south; even numbers indicate east-west routes.

• • • • • • • • • • • • • • • • • • • • • • • • • •

**To remember which exit to take,** watch the small exit panels on the top of road signs. The exit numbers count up or down to your exit.

• • • • • • • • • • • • • • • • • • • • • • • • • •

**To determine whether your exit** will be on the right or left side of the road, watch the position of the small panel on top of the road sign. If it's on the right side of the sign, it's a right lane exit ramp; if it's on the left side, it's a left lane exit ramp; if it's in the middle, there will be one exit and the right or left turn will come after you're off the highway.

• • • • • • • • • • • • • • • • • • • • • • • • •

**Keep toll money in a container in your car.**
If you find yourself forgetting your toll money and digging for spare change at the tollbooth, keep a week's worth of toll money in a plastic film container in your car.

• • • • • • • • • • • • • • • • • • • • • • • • •

**Use an electronic tollway pass.** Purchase an electronic pass (available in most states with toll roads) and you won't need money to physically pay the toll. The electronic pass responder is taped to your windshield near your rearview mirror and an initial fee is charged to your credit card. As you drive through a toll booth, there's no need to stop. An electric eye is triggered and the toll is automatically deducted from your account. When the money in your account is reduced to a certain set level, another charge is made to your credit card. Contact your state motor vehicle department to see if this service is available on your toll roads.

• • • • • • • • • • • • • • • • • • • • • • • • •

# Traveling memories

**Take along pre-addressed labels** when traveling to make sure you remember to send a postcard to everyone. You'll know at a glance which people you still need to write.

- - - - - - - - - - - - - - - - - - - - - - - -

**Write thank-you notes while traveling.** On long trips, take cards, stamps and your address book. Write thank-you notes for gifts, dinners and parties to the people you've seen on your trip. No one will be forgotten, the details will be fresh in your mind and the cards can be mailed in the airport or as soon as you get home.

- - - - - - - - - - - - - - - - - - - - - - - -

**Write down memories from your trip.**
If your memory is sketchy at times, write down a few memories from the trip to relate upon your return home. You might keep a travel book or diary and add postcards, souvenirs or brochures to remind you of where you went and what you did. When you arrive home, you'll have memories to share.

- - - - - - - - - - - - - - - - - - - - -

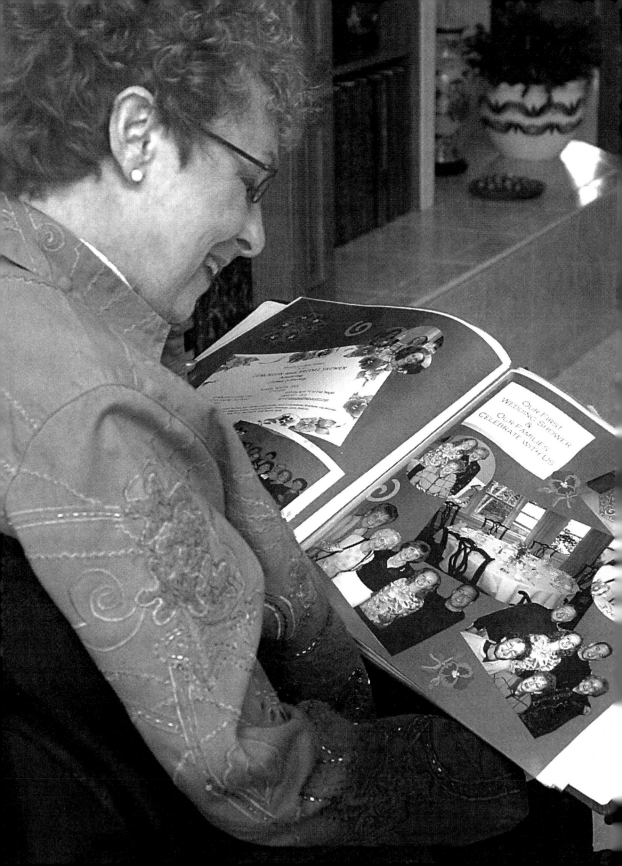

OUR FIRST
WEDDING SHOWER
&
OUR FAMILIE'S
CELEBRATE WITH US

# 9

# having fun

No matter how old you are, you have to have fun and laughter in your life. It improves your physical health along with your mental health and memory. Whether your idea of fun is playing a game, watching a funny movie or visiting and reminiscing, the techniques in this chapter will help you stimulate your mind, stay connected with others and handle the details that enrich your life.

# ASSESSING YOUR NEEDS

**To keep the mind active, it would be helpful to:**

○ Take classes
○ Create art and crafts
○ Listen to or make music
○ Play games
○ Simplify activities
○ Play word games and do puzzles

**To keep memories alive, it would be helpful to:**

○ Reminisce about pleasant events
○ Create a memory box
○ Create a scrapbook
○ Document events, activities and people with photos
○ Make home movies

**To make visiting easier, it would be helpful to:**

○ Keep a photo album with pictures of visitors
○ Keep conversations simple
○ Allow extra time for visits
○ Use short sentences and simple words
○ Close eyes to concentrate
○ Save and reread greeting cards
○ Write an annual birthday letter

**To enjoy leisure activities, it would be helpful to:**

○ Create a personal TV guide
○ Watch videos about a familiar place
○ Subscribe to a movie subscription service
○ Listen to music
○ Listen to books on tape

**To organize holidays and celebrations, it would be helpful to:**

○ Wrap presents in different colors
○ Label and store decorations by season and room
○ Delegate holiday responsibilities
○ Plan ahead for holiday entertaining

**To enjoy the outdoors, it would be helpful to:**

○ Visit a neighborhood park
○ Walk on a bicycle path

# Keeping your mind active

**Take classes.** Universities and colleges often offer free classes for the elderly. (Check with the school to determine if you're old enough to qualify.) Learning new things is a wonderful way to keep your mind and memory operating in peak condition.

• • • • • • • • • • • • • • • • • • • • • • • • • • • •

**Create art.** Remember when you were young how much you enjoyed coloring, painting, modeling clay and other art activities. Get out the crayons, paints and clay and enjoy these activities again. It will be fun and will keep those synapses snapping.

• • • • • • • • • • • • • • • • • • • • • • • • • • • •

**Make music.** Hum along with the radio, sing favorite melodies or play a musical instrument. Not only will you exercise pathways in your brain, you may just attract a group of admirers to interact with.

• • • • • • • • • • • • • • • • • • • • • • • • • • • •

**Play games.** Make time for fun. Do jigsaw puzzles, play Checkers or card games (War, Blackjack, Rummy, Cribbage, etc.) or use picture cards to play Concentration. Playing games will stimulate thinking and problem solving.

• • • • • • • • • • • • • • • • • • • • • • • • • • • •

**Simplify favorite activities.** If your memory makes it difficult to continue favorite activities, scale back to a level you can handle. For example, if you used to do the *New York Times* crossword puzzle, get easier crossword puzzles. Read short stories instead of a whole book. Adjust the rules to favorite games (e.g., when playing Scrabble, allow the use of proper names). Don't give up a favorite pastime; just create a simpler version.

**Keep mentally fit.** Word games, puzzles and problem solving are fun ways to learn new things and keep your mind sharp. Aerobics of the Mind Mental Fitness Cards by Marge Engelman contain 100 activities designed for individuals and small groups of all ages to exercise the brain and improve memory. About $19. Attainment Company, Inc., PO Box 930160, Verona, WI 53953-0160; 800-327-4269; fax 800-942-3865; www.attainmentcompany.com.

# Encouraging memories

**Reminisce about pleasant events** to keep memories alive. Magazines and picture books about country life, babies, animals or another favorite topics can be a catalyst for conversation. Bridal magazines and cookbooks may also be enjoyable.

**Create a memory box.** Decorate a medium-size box with the word "Memories" on the outside. Put photographs, newspaper clippings, mementos of trips and art projects from children and grandchildren inside. A stroll in the memory box will help keep your memories fresh and provide a wonderful opportunity for sharing time with loved ones.

• • • • • • • • • • • • • • • • • • • • • • • •

**Purchase a large scrapbook** and when special days or events roll around, fill a page or two with anecdotes, best wishes, drawings and pictures. The book will be a permanent record of precious times and provide food for happy memories and conversation far in the future.

• • • • • • • • • • • • • • • • • • • • • • • •

**Carry a digital or disposable camera.** A great way to remember special moments is to carry a digital or disposable camera. Tuck it in your purse or pocket so it's always available to capture those unexpected, magical moments. Take pictures at the grocery store, department store, library, car wash, park and so forth. Place them in a photo album or scrapbook so you and others can relive special moments over and over.

• • • • • • • • • • • • • • • • • • • • • • • •

**Make home movies.** Use your video camera to take movies of your family, home and neighborhood. This is a great way to spend time with your family and keep everyone involved in each other's lives.

• • • • • • • • • • • • • • • • • • • • • • • •

# Visiting

**Arrange for visits with family and friends.**
To refresh your memory about each visitor, keep a small photo album that includes a photo of each person along with information about where they work or go to school, their pets, hobbies, children or grandchildren, home and so forth. Ask your visitors questions about their lives and they will do most of the talking, while thinking of you as an amazing conversationalist. Share photographs and stories of your connections and times together. Humorous anecdotes, pearls of wisdom and favorite memories will keep your mind active and memories alive.

**Keep your conversations simple.** When possible, eliminate distractions before trying to communicate. Make eye contact. Position yourself to give or get undivided attention.

**Give yourself extra time** even for the simplest of interactions. If you are easily flustered, stay calm and be patient. Take your time and say what you want to say. In return, be patient and wait for answers.

**Use short sentences and simple words.** If you have trouble finding the right word, speak in simple everyday language. Your listener will likely not notice.

**Close your eyes to concentrate.** This reduces your tension while the other person waits for your next word and eliminates other environmental distractions, allowing you to concentrate better. If you're talking while walking, stop for a moment before closing your eyes. Remember to open your eyes again before you resume walking!

• • • • • • • • • • • • • • • • • • • • • • • • • • •

**Save greeting cards** and reread them when you visit, embellishing with shared stories and memories.

• • • • • • • • • • • • • • • • • • • • • • • • • • •

**Write an annual birthday letter** filled not only with reflections of the year gone by, but also with memories of happy times, shared friends, interests, accomplishments and beloved personality traits. Many happy hours can be passed sharing these letters.

## Entertainment

**Create your own TV guide.** If you have difficulty remembering the time of favorite television programs, make a TV guide that lists in words and pictures the program, channel number and time slot for each day of the week. Post this list of programs next to the TV or favorite chair, perhaps in a stand-up picture frame like in hotels. To make a remote control easier to use, clearly identify important buttons such as on/off and channel changer.

• • • • • • • • • • • • • • • • • • • • • • • • • • •

**Watching videos about a familiar place** or time or some place you'd like to revisit can keep your memory fresh. Rent videos or borrow free videos from the library. Some libraries and video stores (storefront and online) even deliver to your door.

• • • • • • • • • • • • • • • • • • • • • • • • •

**Video subscription services** offer mail delivery and pick-up. If you tend to forget video rentals and late charges pile up, sign up for a subscription service that offers unlimited rentals you can keep as long as you want. Blockbuster, Wal-Mart and Netflix (www.netflix. com) all have plans. Monthly rates run $15.50–30.

• • • • • • • • • • • • • • • • • • • • • • • • •

**Listen to music.** Listening to your favorite music can stimulate your memory and help you relax. Listening to music associated with a particular era (e.g., Big Band) might stir up memories of times when you first heard the music. Buy your favorite music on tape or CD, or borrow music from the library.

• • • • • • • • • • • • • • • • • • • • • • • • •

**Listen to books on tape.** Keep your mind active by listening to books on tape in your car, while working around the house or when out for a walk. For people who have lost the ability to read, consult with your local librarian about the "Talking Book Program," funded by the state and federal government at no cost to the individual.

• • • • • • • • • • • • • • • • • • • • • • • • •

# Holidays

**Wrap each person's gifts** in a different colored paper. You may want to keep a master list of whose gifts are wrapped in which paper. The gifts will be easier to distribute and you won't need name tags.

• • • • • • • • • • • • • • • • • • • • • • •

**Organize holiday decorations** by season and room. To make it easier to remember where all your holiday decorations are, box all the decorations for one room or location together. Label each box with the holiday or season and the room where it belongs. Large objects or stuffed figures too big for boxes can be labeled with a tag indicating the location. If you remove knickknacks, family photos and other personal items during the holiday season, pack these into the empty decoration boxes for that room.

• • • • • • • • • • • • • • • • • • • • • • •

**Delegate holiday responsibilities.** When everyone comes for a holiday dinner, you need to remember many details. Ease the strain on your mind by delegating some responsibility to family members or relatives. They can set the table, place napkins, arrange place cards, fill water glasses and even keep the children occupied in a productive way.

• • • • • • • • • • • • • • • • • • • • • • •

**Plan ahead for holiday entertaining.** To enjoy holiday entertaining more, do as much as you can before your guests arrive. Get out all the serving pieces and utensils, write to-do lists and stick notes on the buffet table where you want everything to go. Doing so will help you remember all the details and make it easier for others to help you.

## The great outdoors

**A trip to the neighborhood park,** pond or woods can be both a stimulating and relaxing outing. The colorful natural surroundings, as well as the activity of birds, animals and children playing, can increase brain activity, capture interest and bring many hours of pleasure.

· · · · · · · · · · · · · · · · · · · · · · · · · · ·

**Walking a bicycle path** is a wonderful way to get fresh air and exercise. These paths have fewer intersections than sidewalks and tend to loop around parks and ponds, making it easier to remember the way home.

· · · · · · · · · · · · · · · · · · · · · · · · · · ·

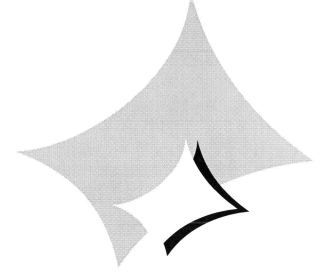

# about the author

Shelley Peterman Schwarz and her husband, Dave, live in Madison, Wisconsin. They've been married since 1969 and are enjoying being the parents of two adult children, Jamie and Andrew, and grandparents to Jamie's little girl, Jordan. Jamie and her husband, David, live and work in Chicago. Andrew and his wife, Ronit, live in Tucson where Andrew is in graduate school at the University of Arizona.

At the time of her multiple sclerosis (MS) diagnosis in 1979, Shelley was working part-time as a teacher of the Deaf. Two years later, due to the effects of progressive MS, she retired. In 1985, when a story she wrote appeared in *Inside MS,* the magazine of the National Multiple Sclerosis Society, a new career was born. Since then Shelley has published more than 450 articles and received numerous awards, including the Mother of the Year from the Wisconsin Chapter of the National MS Society and the Spirit of the American Woman Award from JC Penney. She was also named a Woman of Distinction by the YWCA.

Shelley's nationally syndicated "Making Life Easier" column appears in newspapers and magazines internationally, including *SpeciaLiving, Inside MS, Real Living with MS, Arthritis Today* and *Humana Active Outlook.* Her tips are available on numerous Web sites as well. In 1997 the National Arthritis Foundation, Inc., commissioned Shelley to write *250 Tips for Making Life with Arthritis Easier* based on her "Making Life Easier" column. More Making Life Easier books followed:

- *Dressing Tips and Clothing Resources for Making Life Easier* (Attainment Company, 2000)

- *Multiple Sclerosis: 300 Tips for Making Life Easier* (Demos Medical Publishing, 1999, 2005)

- *Parkinson's Disease: 300 Tips for Making Life Easier* (Demos Medical Publishing, 2002, 2005)

- *Organizing Your IEPs* (Individualized Educational Plans for special education students) (Attainment Company, 2005)

- *Memory Tips for Making Life Easier* (Attainment Company, 2006)

Shelley's words and stories also appear in the following books:

- *Jewish Mothers Tell Their Stories: Acts of Love and Courage* (The Haworth Press, Inc., 2000)

- *A Second Chicken Soup for the Woman's Soul*
  (Health Communications, Inc., 1998)
- *Amazingly Simple Lessons We Learned After 50*
  (M. Evans and Co. Inc., 2001)

In 1995 Shelley self-published *Blooming Where You're Planted: Stories from the Heart.* The previously published essays in this book chronicle her journey of change and self-discovery following her MS diagnosis.

Shelley's philosophy of life is to find solutions to whatever problems she faces and to help others do the same. As a professional speaker, she gives motivational and inspirational keynotes and workshops that help audiences see challenges in their lives as opportunities for personal growth. She shares her message of hope and teaches audiences how to "bloom wherever they're planted."

Visit www.MeetingLifesChallenges.com to contact Shelley, subscribe to her free e-zine, read her blog and personal essays or learn about her teleclasses.